I love to find a book that is important for the NOW season of life that we are journeying through in the earth realm. Being involved in the prayer movement for 20 years or so, I love when I run across a new, creative tool that will help in motivating people to believe in the miracle of prayer. *A Healing Touch* by Melanie Hemry accomplishes both of those quests. Not only is this one of the most enjoyable books that I have read in a very long time, but the HEART CHECK sheet at the end of each chapter is likened to a physical examination of the spirit of man. This will allow us to be "fit" and prepared for the future ahead. *"A man's spirit sustains him in sickness"* (Proverbs 18:14 NIV), and Melanie in *A Healing Touch* makes sure that our spirits are touched and more alive at the end of the book than when we first began reading!

—**Chuck D. Pierce**
President, Glory of Zion International, Inc.
Vice President, Global Harvest Ministries

Melanie Hemry crosses the boundaries between medical healing and spiritual healing—a boundary that is all too often neglected. Her story is a humble reminder that what we are going through at this point in our lives may be no more than a time of refinement that is preparing us for the true task God has planned for us. Melanie offers practical tips on how to best know whether we're staying on that course that God has outlined for us—a set of check points to help us reassess where we stand in regards to the Lord's will for our life. *A Healing Touch* is a perfect guideline for either individual study or group fellowship.

—**David Holland, M.D.**
Physician, Author, Television Guest

I'd like to introduce you to a book by Melanie Hemry called *A Healing Touch*. What I love about it is that, as a registered nurse, Melanie knows about physical healing but she's also a wonderful Christian who understands spiritual healing.

I really enjoyed the chapter about finishing the course. It's amazing. Here you have nurses running in a race, and a guy just drops dead right in front of them—talk about being in the right place at the right time! Melanie has had many experiences that will bless you, and I hope her book ministers as much to you as it ministered to me.

Melanie has been such a blessing to my ministry over the years. She's one of the finest authors we've had the opportunity to work with. She's written many articles for my ministry, and we have been pleased with every one.

So, sit down and get yourself a cup of coffee because, not only are you about to read a good book about healing, but you are also about to be inspired to reach out and spiritually touch a person for God. After this book, you'll understand why God called Melanie Hemry to minister to us in this matter. Enjoy!

—**Dr. Jesse Duplantis**
Jessie Duplantis Ministries

Those of us in the field of medicine have many opportunities to witness miraculous events. When one is tuned into these events and the reason for them, like Melanie Hemry has been for many years, it can make for some very revealing reading that can inspire each of us to capitalize on the power of prayer.

—**Benjamin Carson, M.D.**
Director of Pediatric Neurosurgery
John Hopkins Hospital
Author, *Gifted Hands, Think Big,* and *The Big Picture*

I love Melanie Hemry's book, *A Healing Touch*! I devoured it and couldn't put it down. I did not expect it to challenge and change me as it did. What a surprise to realize that this was more than a great book. It is a book of parables with a Heart Check key to each one. Chapter by chapter, I was led into a deeper place in God, hungry for MORE. I became eager to be used by Him in prayer and in my daily life. I was changed in a significant way, not just *wishing* I could know Him and be used by Him, but actually doing it! I look forward to sharing *A Healing Touch* with others.

—**Rebecca Goen Stough, M.D.**

Melanie has the unique gift to serve in the healing of people both physically and spiritually. *A Healing Touch* reminds me that God has put us all in a mission field and we have to allow Him to use us in miraculous ways—and all through the power of prayer! Her personal nursing stories have been an inspiration to me as I work and minister in the Hollywood entertainment industry mission field. Thanks, Melanie!

—**Karen Covell**
Director of the Hollywood Prayer Network
TV Producer, and Author, *The Day I Met God*
and *How to Talk about Jesus without Freaking Out*

This is a noisy world with many loud voices. Melanie has reminded us that only God's voice brings life! Through her medical experiences, gift of writing, humor, and personal encounters with God, she has powerfully challenged all of us to hear Him daily for ourselves. Besides all that, it's fun to read! It's like ER with godly insight!

—**Dr. John Benefiel**
Chairman, Oklahoma Apostolic Prayer Network
Founder and Senior Pastor, Church on the Rock,
Oklahoma City, OK

a Healing TOUCH

DEDICATION

To my daughters, Heather and Lauren,
you are God's greatest gift to me and the reason
I will praise Him all my days.

a Healing TOUCH

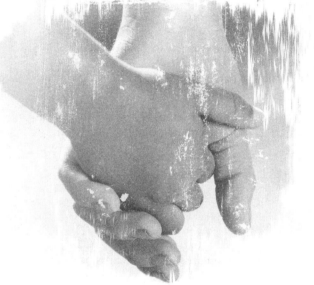

THE POWER OF PRAYER

MELANIE HEMRY

WHITAKER
HOUSE

A HEALING TOUCH:
The Power of Prayer

For speaking engagements, please contact the author through:
www.melaniehemry.com

ISBN-13: 978-0-88368-780-2 • ISBN-10: 0-88368-780-1
Printed in the United States of America
© 2006 by Melanie Hemry

1030 Hunt Valley Circle
New Kensington, PA 15068
www.whitakerhouse.com

Library of Congress Cataloging-in-Publication Data
Hemry, Melanie, 1949–
A healing touch : the power of prayer / Melanie Hemry.
p. cm.
Summary: "An introduction to intercessory prayer, based on the author's experiences"—Provided by publisher.
ISBN-13: 978-0-88368-780-2 (trade pbk. : alk. paper)
ISBN-10: 0-88368-780-1 (trade pbk. : alk. paper)
1. Intercessory prayer—Christianity. 2. Hemry, Melanie, 1949– I. Title.
BV210.3.H46 2006
248.3'2—dc22   2006008970

2 3 4 5 6 7 8 9 10 11 12 13 14 ᴜᴜ 17 16 15 14 13 12 11 10 09 08

FOREWORD

I first met Melanie Hemry at a beginning writer's workshop I attended in the 1980s. Fresh from a sixteen-year career in nursing, much of that time spent in critical care, Melanie was full of vision and talent. While the rest of us were still working on submissions, her writing career took off early when she won the prestigious national Guideposts Writing Contest and then began to establish a solid career as a ghostwriter, serving pastors and leaders in the body of Christ.

Truly one of the best true-life drama writers in the industry, Melanie has a depth of spiritual understanding and experience that matches her medical expertise and skill with words. I greatly admire her as a writer, friend, and fellow sojourner in the spiritual life. That's why I'm so honored to recommend her book to you.

In *A Healing Touch: The Power of Prayer,* she combines what she knows best—her medical background and heart for God, people, and ministry—to create a book full of compelling stories and valuable instruction.

A Healing Touch will challenge you, inspire you, and equip you to make a difference in a hurting world. Gone are the days when playing church or being a nominal believer was enough. We live in a time of tremendous uncertainty that offers enormous opportunities for the kingdom of God. *A Healing Touch* is a book that will prepare you to join God in His search-and-rescue mission to a critically wounded world.

—*Cheri Fuller*
Author and Motivational Speaker

TABLE OF CONTENTS

CHAPTER ONE

COMING OF AGE

*When I was a child, I talked like a child, I thought like
a child, I reasoned like a child. When I became a man,
I put childish ways behind me.*
—1 Corinthians 13:11

The sound of moaning respirators and the putrid smell of burned flesh assailed me as I pushed my way through the double doors into the intensive care unit that afternoon. Before the doors shut behind me, I knew I was in for a hard shift. Room ten, our only isolation area, held a fresh burn patient. One nurse would spend the evening in that room. Following report, I walked past the cubicles, mentally assessing the unit.

*One burn patient. One patient with acute congestive heart fail-
ure. One patient with an acute cardiac infarction. One patient with
cardiac arrhythmia admitted for cardioversion. Five fresh open-heart
surgery patients due out of recovery anytime.*

I rubbed sweaty palms against the soft white material of my uniform. Until recently, I had worked on a medical-surgical ward with forty patients. But those patients hadn't been critical. Many had been *terminal*, and many had died. But those deaths were usually the result of the aging process, or chronic long-term illness. Critical patients—those with a sudden, usually unexpected, catastrophic event—were admitted to the intensive care unit.

Well, I wanted a new challenge, I reminded myself as I handed out assignments. I'd never felt the weight of life and death rest on me so heavily. My orientation to critical care was over; for the first time, I was Team Leader in charge.

There were rites-of-passage that critical care nurses had to navigate in order to be accepted by the doctors and other nurses. Whatever mild testing I'd endured as a staff nurse the past months was nothing compared to the scrutiny and testing I would endure to win acceptance as Team Leader. I watched the seasoned nurses work and knew that no matter what happened in the next eight hours, I could count on one thing.

I was on my own.

Two hours later the cardiovascular surgeon on call arrived to check the five new open-heart patients before going home for the evening. I handed him the chart for the patient in room three.

"His blood pressure has dropped slowly and steadily since he arrived from recovery," I reported. "I've given him extra IV fluids and a unit of blood to bring up his volume, but the recovery each time is temporary. I'm concerned that he might have tamponade."

I hesitated to even say the word *tamponade.* One of the deadliest complications of heart surgery, it occurred when blood pooled around the heart until finally, it stopped beating. The condition was hard to recognize, and once established, could only be reversed by surgery.

The surgeon shot questions at me like bullets from a firing squad, and then examined the man, listening for long minutes to his heart sounds.

"He's just volume depleted," the doctor said. "Give him another unit of blood and a 1,000cc bottle of fluid."

The blood and extra fluid pumped his blood pressure up to a healthy 130/70. His cheeks pinked up, and he looked better than he had since surgery. I checked the other patients, then donned a gown, mask, and gloves to help with the burn patient.

Later, I read the nurses' notes lying neatly on the bedside table in room three. None of the vital signs leapt off the paper, waving a red flag at me. His blood pressure had drifted back down, urine output had slowed considerably, and there'd been very little drainage from the chest tubes. I'd seen dozens of patients like him in the past month. So why was my mouth dry and my stomach tied in a knot? And *why* did I feel a sense of doom?

It's what you know after you know it all that counts.
—Anonymous

Probably just nervous about my first shift as Team Leader, I thought, picking up one of the man's chest tubes that drained blood from the surgical area to "milk" it. Even as I tried, I knew it was a useless gesture. Milking the chest tubes moved blood clots down the tube and kept them open and draining. I'd assigned one of the most experienced nurses in the unit to this patient. She'd milked the tubes so long her fingers were red and swollen. If there was a blood clot high in that chest tube, it wasn't for her lack of attention.

Something was wrong. But how could I explain a sense of doom arising from somewhere in my gut to a cocky young cardiovascular surgeon who'd spent twelve years learning what he knew? He had the education, and he had the initials—a long line of them—trailing his name on a starched white lab coat. I could just imagine what he'd say if I called him *again* on Friday evening. *Something's wrong all right! Something's wrong with the nurse left in charge!*

If one of the more experienced nurses phoned him, he might not like it, but he'd listen seriously to what she said. And he *might* consider taking this man back to surgery.

Maybe she'll call him for me, I thought, glancing at one of the older nurses. She read my face like the Sunday newspaper.

"Not on your life," she said, turning on her heel and walking away.

I tried not to take it personally. We all wanted the same thing: for these patients to make it out of here alive. But critical care nurses are very protective of their patients. The nurses on duty that evening needed to know what I'd do when they *weren't* around. That's the only way they could relax and trust me on their day off. Their expressions read, "No leaning allowed!" If I didn't measure up, my career in critical care would be short.

I dialed the doctor's phone number.

"Dr. Roberts*," he barked. I gave him a quick report on the patient in room three.

"Why don't you go back to floor duty where you belong?" he asked, sarcasm dripping off each word. "Whatever possessed you to think you could take care of critically ill patients? You have no business in that unit. I suppose we got stuck with you because the job corps didn't want you. Now listen to me, and listen carefully. Don't you dare call me back tonight."

A dial tone sounded in my ear. *He hung up on me!*

---

* Indicates name has been changed.

I stood still, blushing to the roots of my hair. Looking around, I saw that every nurse in the unit had positioned herself to hear my end of the conversation. The looks on their faces let me know that they agreed in spades with whatever he had said.

It's not enough to know how to treat these patients, their lifted eyebrows and pointed stares seemed to say, *if you can't deal with prima donna doctors and earn their respect—you're history!*

I set up eight o'clock meds and helped with vital signs. Then I walked over to the patient in bed three.

"How are you feeling?" I asked, rubbing my hand over his arm. His skin felt cold and clammy.

"Like I've been run over by a Mac truck," he said with a crooked smile. "I feel so *weak.*"

> *G*od offers a tough love that turns us into sweeter and stronger persons.
> —*Robert Harold Shuller*

We made small talk while I tried to figure out what to do. Should I pursue getting him back to surgery? I might as well face facts. I'd never actually *seen* a case of tamponade. It was a rare complication, and I'd only read about it in a textbook.

If I was wrong about him having tamponade, and someone believed me, the patient would endure a second surgery unnecessarily. As for me—I'd lose my career in critical care.

But if the man *did* have tamponade, and I didn't pursue help for him, he would die.

Again I felt that sense of doom. I didn't have any good choices.

Career or death.

Death seemed so much more...permanent.

I checked the patient's chart. Dr. Burns*, the senior partner of Dr. Robert's group had done the surgery. If I tried to call him on his night off, the answering service would simply transfer the call to Dr. Roberts. Besides, Dr. Burns and his wife, Susan,* were well known for their dinner parties. Most likely they were entertaining now.

Susan—his wife! Now there was an idea. Surely Susan's friends could get past the answering service. *Kiss your career good-bye*, I thought as I dialed Dr. Burn's number.

"Dr. Burns' residence," the answering service operator said.

"I'd like to speak to Susan, please."

"Hello?" Susan asked.

"Hi, Susan. I'm the Team Leader at the CCU. I've got a real concern about one of Dr. Burns' patients. I'm sorry I went around your answering service, but I really need to speak to Dr. Burns," I said. Then rushed to add, "It's urgent!"

A long silence followed, and I heard the tinkling of glasses and murmured conversation in the background. *Oh Lord, they're having a party.*

"Hold on," she said at last, "I'll get him."

"Yes?" Dr. Burns snapped when he came on the line.

"I'm concerned about one of your patients," I said, after identifying myself. I outlined the man's condition, giving him all the pertinent information.

"Have you called Dr. Roberts?"

"Yes, I've spoken to him several times, and he's been here to examine the patient."

"And what does *he* say?"

18

"That it's low blood volume."

"And you think its tamponade because…?"

"I admit that his blood pressure isn't *that* low, and his urine output is low, but still within acceptable limits…."

"So his vital signs are indicative of low blood volume?" he interrupted.

"Yes, sir."

"Then why did you call me?"

"Because while his vital signs might reflect low blood volume, they could also be early warning signs of tamponade."

I took a deep breath. The silence on the other end of the line was deafening. I was getting nowhere. I may as well lay it all on the line.

"And…well…I have this sickening feeling in my gut that this man is going to die unless he goes back to surgery."

"Your gut?"

"Yes, sir, my gut."

Now it was Dr. Burns' turn to sigh. "I'll be there in a few minutes."

The double door of the intensive care unit flew backward in unleashed fury a few minutes later. I gasped when I looked up. There was Dr. Burns…*and Dr. Roberts!*

Somehow it had never occurred to me that he would bring Dr. Roberts. His face turned dull red when he saw me, and he flashed a murderous look my way. His fury seemed to fill every molecule of space in the room.

Trembling, I picked up the chart and followed them to the patient's bedside. Dr. Burns seemed resigned and weary. Dr. Roberts' rage was about as contained as an oil field fire. Only the presence of his senior partner held him back. His looks let me know that I would pay—dearly—for putting him in this situation.

"I called in the surgical staff before I left home," Dr. Burns said, slowly letting each word have its full impact. "They're waiting for us now." He spoke to the patient for a few minutes, and then he and Dr. Roberts left to go scrub for the surgery. He paused in the doorway and looked back at me.

"You'd better be right," Dr. Burns said.

Everyone was subdued after we got the patient to surgery. It felt like the calm before a storm. The administrator-on-call stopped by and asked me to check a patient on the eighth floor. Afterward, I was about to step on the elevator when I heard my name announced over the hospital speaker system.

> *Maturity is the stage where the whole life has been brought under the control of God.*
>
> —Oswald Chambers

"Report to surgery at once!"

I felt physically sick when the elevator bounced to a stop on the second floor. I pushed my way into the icy halls of surgery and saw a nurse waiting for me.

"Dr. Burns wants you in there *now*," she said.

"But I'm not scrubbed…"

"Just don't touch anything," she ordered, shoving me inside the operating suite.

Dr. Burns glanced at me over his glasses, and then ignored my presence. Dr. Roberts never looked my way. Long minutes passed as I listened to the whir of the respirator, the rhythmic pumping of the heart-lung machine, and the gentle clinking of surgical instruments. I could feel my heart pounding a staccato rhythm in my throat.

"This patient had tamponade," Dr. Burns said softly while he tied a suture. "He would have died if we hadn't operated on him when we did."

I let out a long, slow breath and started backing out of the room.

"Wait!" Dr. Burns ordered. "My partner has something he wants to say to you."

"You were right," Dr. Roberts mumbled behind his surgical mask, never looking up.

"Thank you," I said, turning to leave.

"Not so fast," Dr. Burns said. "There is one more thing Dr. Roberts wants to say to you."

I stopped and waited.

Silence.

Minutes passed while every person in the room looked uncomfortable. Finally, I broke the silence.

"It doesn't matter…"

"Oh, but it *does* matter," Dr. Burns insisted. "Dr. Roberts has something very important to say to you. Don't you?"

Silence.

"Say it!" Dr. Burns insisted.

Silence.

"I told you to say it!"

Dr. Roberts' face flushed a deep red. Finally, he choked out two words.

"Happy birthday."

Happy birthday?

I'd forgotten that it was my birthday. They must have seen

my birthday cake—still uncut—in the break room. None of us had had time for a break all evening. The white icing sported blue letters. "Happy Birthday, Melanie."

I was twenty-one years old.

I'd come of age.

Today, the church is facing her own coming-of-age crisis: Terrorist attacks, biological warfare, AIDS, school massacres, child abuse, domestic violence, drive-by shootings, war, and genocide.

We have been handed the responsibility of nursing a critically wounded world. That same world is silently watching to see if the church has the answer. After two thousand years, one thing is clearly unchanged.

The world *still* needs a Savior.

Will they find Him…in *you*?

God appoints our graces to be nurses to other men's weaknesses.
—Henry Ward Beecher

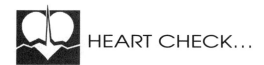 HEART CHECK...

You may never be tested by fire in the intensive care unit, but if you accept the call to provide *A Healing Touch* for a hurting world, at some point you may face your own coming-of-age experience. Whether through prayer, intercession, or a physical response, these experiences reveal just what we're willing to risk in order to save a life.

√ **What am I willing to risk?**
- Sleep, if God needs someone to pray during the night watch?
- Time, if God asks me to intervene?
- Reputation, if I'm misunderstood?
- What am I willing to put on the altar?

One of the first ways to begin training for *A Healing Touch* is to pay attention to gentle nudges from God. In the story you just read, that nudge was no more than a gut feeling. Because God's ways are higher than ours, His nudges don't always make sense to the natural mind. Will there be times when what you thought was a nudge from God was really your own misplaced idea? Absolutely! But you will never learn the difference unless you pay attention to those quiet spiritual directions and pray, asking God to lead you.

√ **What nudges have I ignored?**
- The best way to learn to recognize God's voice is to get to know Him. To know His voice, recognize His whispers, and feel His heart. As believers, we'll have all of eternity to explore the different facets of God. Why not begin now?

√ I purpose in my heart to know Him.

- The best way to know God is through His Word. Buy *The One Year Bible*, which is arranged in 365 daily readings. One year from now you'll know Him from Genesis to Revelation. Next year you can switch to a different translation of the same Bible. Day by day and year by year, you'll know Him more deeply.

- Cultivate communication. Greet God each morning and talk to Him as you would a friend—all through the day. God is listening, and since we're made in His image, we like a lot of the same things. Like saying, "I love you!" for no reason.

- Ask God to show you a hurting world through His eyes.

- Move your faith from your head to your heart by reaffirming that you need a savior. Search your heart and make sure you aren't relying on your church affiliation, your traditions, or your own good deeds instead of the finished work of the cross.

Heavenly Father, forgive me for everything in my life that has hurt You and our relationship. I am willing to provide a healing touch for a hurting world. Train me to give intensive care in these critical times. Since Jesus risked everything for me, help me to risk those things You ask of me in order to save lives. Teach me to recognize and respond to Your gentle nudges. Above all, help me to know You now and for all eternity. I ask this in Jesus' name. Amen.

CHAPTER TWO

WAITING ON GOD

In the morning, O LORD, you hear my voice; in the morning
I lay my requests before you and wait in expectation.
—Psalm 5:3

When I awoke the morning after my coming-of-age experience in nursing, I moaned as I rolled out of bed. I didn't *feel* twenty-one. I felt *old*. I felt older than Abraham. I felt older than Methuselah. I felt like I'd already seen too much in twenty-one years. But nursing, especially intensive care nursing, makes you grow up hard and fast. When I crawled into bed that night, I asked myself for the hundredth time, *Why am I doing this?*

I'd always dreamed of being a writer, but no one in my family had gone to college and there simply wasn't enough money for my parents to send me. In my desperate desire for a college education, I accepted a part-time job as a nursing assistant at a local hospital. I naively believed I could save enough money to put myself through college while earning minimum wage. After working half days at the hospital during high school, I was offered a partial college scholarship—in nursing.

My thoughts drifted back to my senior year. *What should I do?* I wondered as my high school graduation loomed on the horizon. *I want to be a writer, not a nurse. But this scholarship is the only way I see to go to college.* Didn't the Bible promise that if we asked God for wisdom, He'd give it to us?

This qualifies, I thought. *I need God's wisdom now.*

"Father," I prayed, "I need wisdom. You know I've made plans for my life—plans to go to college and be a writer. Now, I've been given this scholarship in nursing. I guess it's time I ask *You*—what do You want me to do with my life?"

I listened for an answer while I pulled on my white uniform and dressed for work. "Well, Lord?" I asked impatiently, while driving to the hospital. After lunch, I made a quick change and rushed to my first class.

"Lord...*are You there?*" I asked, pulling my books from the locker.

> *G*od has given man one tongue and two ears that we may hear twice as much as we speak.
>
> —*Anonymous*

At five o'clock I drove home and helped my mother start dinner. Later, with my homework spread across the kitchen table, I strummed my fingers on the tabletop and listened for God's answer.

Nothing.

I had a babysitting job that evening that kept me running until I dropped into bed late that night. I pulled myself out of bed the next morning at six and talked to God while I dressed for work. "Lord, I *really* want Your will for my life, but I can't be held responsible for something I don't know. When are You going to show me what to do?" I tugged on my white hose, finished dressing, grabbed a biscuit from the breakfast table, and rushed to work.

I fed one of my patients breakfast then went to gather clean linens for her bed. I'd just opened the linen closet door when I heard a roar and the sound of a chair being kicked across the room. I threw myself in the linen closet and slammed the door. One of the doctors had a horrible temper. *He must have bumped his leg against the hand crank on one of our old hospital beds again,* I thought. I huddled in the dark listening as he raged and cursed, knocking furniture around. *Lord, please don't call me to this.*

Weeks flew by in a busy haze of senior pictures, printing graduation announcements, dates, and my senior prom. When would I hear from God?

> *T*he first duty of love is to listen.
> —Paul Johanes Oskar Tillich

One night I lay in bed thumbing through my Bible. I turned to Psalm 25 and began to read. The fifth verse seemed to leap off the paper. *"Lead me in Your truth and teach me, for You are the God of my salvation; on You I wait all the day"* (NKJV).

Yeah, Lord, I'm waiting.

A few minutes later Psalm 27:14 seemed to light up on the page. *"Wait for the LORD; be strong and let your heart take courage; yes, wait for the LORD"* (NASB).

The Bible talks a lot about waiting, doesn't it?

I read a few more chapters and saw, *"Be still, and know that I am God"* (Psalm 46:10).

I paused. Those psalms seemed to be speaking to me. Be *still,* and *wait.*

Suddenly I blushed. What had I been thinking? I had asked the God of the universe for direction, but I hadn't sat still to wait on a reply. I'd talked to Him on the run to work, whispered a sentence between classes, and moved ahead with my life at the speed of light.

I would have never considered treating a friend that way. If I asked someone a question, I would wait expectantly for an answer. Yet, I'd spoken to God, never waiting for Him to answer. I'd given Him my half-hearted attention while driving through busy traffic, while I talked to patients at work and listened to my teachers at school.

"Father, I'm sorry," I whispered. The phone rang as I said it.

I lay awake late that night. Where in my busy schedule could I make time to *listen* to God?

The next afternoon after school I pulled on a pair of old jeans, sneakers, and my favorite plaid shirt. "I'm going to sit in the pasture," I told Mother, nodding toward the farm at the end of our block.

"The pasture?" my mother asked, raising an eyebrow. "Why?"

"It's the only place I know where I can get quiet enough to hear God's voice. I need to know what He wants me to do with my life."

She looked at me and smiled. "That's a good idea," she said. "Don't worry about helping with supper."

The world seemed alive with promise as I climbed over the barbed-wire fence and strolled to a clump of trees. Black and white cattle stopped chewing to gaze at me. I sat down in the soft spring grass, still moist from a morning rain, and leaned my back against the tree I'd climbed hundreds of times as a child. The sun felt warm on my face as I listened to the swish of the cow's tails swatting flies. The hustle-bustle world suddenly seemed far away and less important than the caterpillar that climbed up my sleeve.

"Well, Lord, here I am," I said, breaking the silence. "Since I became a Christian, I guess I've spent a lot of time telling You what I think…and what I need. I can't say I've ever spent any time giving You a chance to speak to me. But that's why I'm here today. So…I'll just be quiet."

I sat still and waited.

An hour passed, then two. Reluctantly, I climbed back over the fence and walked home. I wasn't any wiser about God's plan for my life, but as I waited on the Lord, something inside me that had been coiled tight began to unwind. I couldn't even give it a name.

> *I*t's just as important to listen to someone with your eyes as it is with your ears.
> —*Martin Buxbaum*

The next afternoon, I rushed home and changed into my jeans. "You're going back to the pasture again?" my mother asked.

I paused at the door. "I'm going every day until I hear from God."

Once again, she nodded her silent approval. A few minutes later, I sank into the soft grass. "I'm back, Lord," I said. "I'm going to be still and wait on You."

A cow tugged at the tender grass near my feet and contemplated my sneakers.

I didn't hear anything from God that day.

Or the next.

Yet, day after day as I waited—quiet and still—my perspective changed. *My* plans, *my* career, *my* school, *my* job, and *my* needs all began to pale in significance to His presence.

Some days it seemed that the Lord drew my attention to magnificent, billowing clouds that formed overhead. Other times my senses danced when He brushed my hair with His breeze, and His sunlight kissed my cheeks.

The world became new and vibrant to me during those hours.

> *G*ive us grace to listen well.
> —John Keble

A butterfly fluttering on a leaf left me breathless. That day, I broke my silence. I didn't mean to do it, but awe of God welled up in me from some place so deep that it couldn't be stopped.

I threw back my head and sang.

I sang hymns.

I sang love songs.

I sang everything that was in my heart.

Afterward, I lay spent in the grass and felt the weight of His presence in every molecule of my being.

This must be how David felt when he was a shepherd, I thought. *All alone with God and the sheep—no wonder he wrote so many songs.*

A week passed, then two.

I could hardly wait to climb that fence each day. The time I spent alone with God became the hub around which the rest of my life turned.

I had just settled against my favorite tree one afternoon when a cow ambled over and looked at me with soft brown eyes. A moment later, God spoke.

God, the Creator of the heaven and earth.

God, who measured the foundation of the world with His hand.

God, in whose presence I had finally learned to wait.

God spoke.

The voice wasn't audible, but it echoed through every cell of my body. Thirty years later, the sound of those words are as real to me as they were that day.

"I am calling you into nursing. In your later years, you will write."

Today, I'm still following those simple instructions from God. I worked as a registered nurse for nearly sixteen years before trading in my stethoscope for a computer and going back to school to begin a second career as a freelance writer.

I'd like to say that I had the wisdom to wait on Him at every crossroads in my life.

Sadly, I did not.

Sadder still are the millions of people who wander aimlessly through their lives never taking the time to know God's plan. Without His plan it is impossible to find our place in the church.

I've had people desperate for God's will ask me, "Do *you* know what God wants me to do?"

"No, I don't. But you can know if you'll learn to listen to God."

Looking around the body of Christ, I believe we are becoming a praying church. We pray all kinds of prayer. We pray petitions. We pray supplications. We pray intercessions. We pray in the Spirit. We pray the Word. We pray thanksgiving.

Then, the moment we stop speaking and God opens His mouth to answer—we walk away.

We may be a praying people.

But we haven't been a listening people,

The people God will use in the critical days ahead will be those who are willing to wait on Him. God is speaking all the time. Is anyone listening?

Will you?

*G*od never comes
to those who do
not wait.
—*Frederick William
Faber*

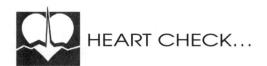 HEART CHECK...

It is no accident that this story appears so early in the book; it is by design. The most important aspect of providing *A Healing Touch* for a wounded world is the ability to hear God's voice. You may not be able to sit in a pasture, but here are some ways you can listen and wait on God:

√ **Practice Silence**

- Even if you begin at five minutes a day, turn off the noise—television, radio, CD player, personal computer, and telephone. Be still and listen.
- Brownbag a lunch and sit in a garden or beside a pond and listen.
- Take an early morning or late evening walk—leaving the Walkman behind.
- Relax in a hot bubble bath and soak your soul and spirit in His presence.
- Sign up for a "Quiet Retreat" where no one speaks.
- Curl up in your favorite chair and meditate on a psalm.

If you still can't silence the noise in your head, play soft worship music and praise Him until the heavy, peaceful silence falls...then *listen.*

Father, teach me to still the noise that bombards my soul each day—all the self talk that jabbers on about what I should be doing with my time and often condemns me. Help me learn to wait patiently while I fine-tune my spirit to Your frequency. Help me learn to listen to You in quiet whispers as You restore my soul. I ask this in Jesus' name. Amen.

CHAPTER THREE

You're Responsible for What You Know

Therefore this generation will be held responsible.
—Luke 11:50

The temperature dropped below zero by mid-afternoon that winter day, and I slid to work on ice-covered streets. We were in a recession. Loosely translated, the average citizen didn't have money for the luxury of doctor visits early in an illness. Each time the economy plunged, the intensive care units burst at the seams. People simply waited too long to seek help.

I'd never encountered a sicker group of patients than the ones who awaited me in the coronary care unit that day. The evening flew by in a blur of exhaustion. I could hardly face the night shift when they arrived at 11 p.m. Already short-staffed, someone had called in sick. There wasn't anyone left to call for help. We'd all given up our days off and added extra shifts to handle the over-load. Yet, when I looked at the handful of people who showed up for the night shift, I wasn't sure it was humanly possible for them to do what had to be done.

The Team Leader's eyes pled with me each time I looked at her. She wanted me to stay and work through the night, but I simply had to rest. Before I finished my report to the evening shift, the emergency room sent up a new burn patient.

"I'll stay until you get the burn patient settled," I said, feeling exhausted and overwhelmed.

We worked furiously until one a.m. Finally, there was a lull. "Sorry," I said, pulling on my coat and gloves, "but I've got to get some sleep."

I was almost out the door when the hospital operator announced, "Doctor A, X-ray!" That code meant that someone had died in X-ray, and they were requesting any doctor in the building to help. Hospital policy required that a coronary care nurse respond as well.

"*Please* respond to that resuscitation before you go," the night nurse begged. I groaned inwardly as I pulled off my coat and gloves. *A few more minutes and I would have been gone!* I thought as I ran out the double doors.

A large man, probably in his fifties, lay dead on an X-ray table. Two other people responded to the call—a fourth year medical student and a doctor. I read the doctor's nametag and realized he was a pathologist.

The two men did CPR while I started an IV. *What is a pathologist doing here at one o'clock in the morning?* I wondered, shoving the first ampoule of sodium bicarbonate into the IV tubing. Then I remembered all the bodies we'd rolled to the morgue in the past few weeks and decided I really didn't want to know.

The patient was in full cardiac arrest. We worked hard to make his heart do something—*anything* but a straight line. We gave adrenaline through a long needle into his heart.

Finally, the heart started fibrillating. He was still dead, but we hoped to convert the useless quivering to regular contractions. We shocked the heart with 400 watts of electricity, then paused a moment to check his rhythm. I glanced at the monitor and saw the large wide contractions indicative of a dying heart pattern. The rhythm, at twenty beats per minute, wasn't pumping blood. Still, it was the first hint of life we'd seen. I pulled a potent cardiac stimulant from the emergency cart, certain the doctor would order a drip.

About that time, he took a good look at the monitor. "PVCs!" he shouted. "Give him a bolus of lidocaine."

The moment he yelled PVCs I knew it would be a long night. *Why didn't I go home at 11:30?* I thought, trying to stifle a sigh.

The doctor misread the cardiac rhythm.

The buck stops here.

—Anonymous motto mounted on the desk of President Harry S. Truman

Certainly this rhythm looked large and wide like PVCs. But by definition a PVC—premature ventricular contraction—was *premature* to the normal rhythm and was considered dangerous. If these were PVCs, the drug he suggested would help.

But *this* rhythm wasn't premature to anything, because there wasn't any other rhythm. This rhythm was all he had going for him. Lidocaine, used to anesthetize the heart and stop PVCs, would put him back into cardiac arrest.

With one singular difference—after the lidocaine there would be no chance of saving him.

I did *not* want to tell this semi-hysterical, totally exhausted medical doctor that he was wrong. But, by law, I had no choice.

Our state law was clear as a bell: You're responsible for what you know!

If a doctor errs in ordering a medication, and the nurse gives the drug *knowing* it is wrong—it is legally considered to be an act of negligence. *In spite of the doctor's order.*

I could not administer that drug.

"Those aren't PVCs," I said quietly. "He's in a dying heart pattern. If we give lidocaine, we'll never get him out of cardiac arrest. He needs another cardiac stimulant."

"*Those are PVCs!*" he shouted, pointing a finger at the cardiac monitor. "Now give him a bolus of lidocaine and start a drip!"

"I'm sorry, I can't do that."

"You *what?*"

"I can't give the lidocaine. I'm responsible for what I know, and I know lidocaine will stop the only heart rhythm he has."

He was enraged. I understood his feelings, but, frankly, pathologists' patients didn't usually have a heartbeat. He probably hadn't seen a cardiac monitor since he left medical school.

He grabbed a two-gram ampoule of lidocaine and handed it to the medical student. "Give this IV push," he ordered.

I shuddered, waiting to see what the medical student would do. That two-gram ampoule was designed to mix in a 500cc bottle of fluid and drip slowly over several hours. Given straight IV push, it would kill an Olympic athlete.

The medical student uncapped the needle and started to shove it into the IV tube.

Dear God.

"Don't give that!" I snapped, countermanding the order. "That's *two grams* of lidocaine in your hand. Even if this man

38

needed lidocaine—which he doesn't—the dose is 50 to 100 milligrams per kilogram of body weight."

He stopped, clearly shaken.

"I told you to *give it*," the doctor ordered.

Once again the medical student moved to administer the drug.

"That drug and that dose are lethal," I said softly. "And it is malpractice."

By now the medical student was sweating.

I felt sorry for him. Glancing around, I felt sorry for all of us. Judging by looks, the only difference between us and the dead man was that we were still standing.

> *R*esponsibility educates.
> —Wendell Phillips

We were on the same team. Death was our enemy. We'd each sworn to fight death and uphold life. We had a common goal. More than rest, more than sleep, more than *anything*, we all wanted this man to live.

We simply couldn't agree on the best way to make that happen.

The doctor, shaking with rage, grabbed the lidocaine. "I'll do it myself," he hissed, glaring at the medical student as though he were a traitor.

A tall man, he lifted the dose toward the light to squeeze air out of the needle.

I turned to leave.

You've done all you can, I assured myself. *You refused to give the drug. You told them both the truth.* I sighed. It was time to go home. There was nothing else for me to do.

But he's going to kill this man, my heart screamed.

You can't kill a corpse, my head reasoned.

The man deserves a chance!

Yeah, well, life isn't fair.

But as I stepped toward the door, a sparkle caught my eye. It was the exam light shining on…a wedding band.

Suddenly, he wasn't just a corpse. He was someone's husband. Probably a father. Someone whose chair would be forever empty at the dinner table. Those gray lifeless lips would never smile again. He would never call, "Merry Christmas!" to those he loved.

Just leave. No one will ever know what happened here tonight.

I would know.

I didn't think; I reacted. Just as he turned to give the medication, I grabbed his arm and jerked it back.

"Don't do this," I begged.

"You're *crazy!*" he screamed. "Let go of my arm."

I didn't.

He raised his arm above my head and tried to shake me loose. I hung on, my feet dangling above the floor.

I wouldn't let go.

Maybe he was too tired to fight. Maybe he thought I really had gone crazy. Maybe my dogged determination made him question his own decision. For whatever reason, he gave up and lay the drug aside. In its place, he picked up a pen and paper. Reading my nametag aloud, he copied it onto the paper.

"I'll have you fired tomorrow," he said, then turned on his heel and walked out of the room.

I can't believe I put my whole career on the line for a corpse.

The medical student jumped when I moved. He was scared.

I didn't blame him.

Following standard resuscitation orders written by the chief of cardiology, I connected an IV drip of one of the most potent cardiac stimulants. Within minutes a normal rhythm marched across the monitor screen.

The man took a shuddering breath on his own. We moved him to a stretcher and ran all the way to intensive care.

I didn't get a call from the medical director the next day. He probably pulled the chart and looked at the rhythm strips I'd posted, though. Then he explained the concept of a dying heart pattern to a weary pathologist who'd seen enough death to last him a lifetime.

I didn't have any illusions that I knew more than that doctor. He had more information packed in his frontal lobe than I would learn in a lifetime. But in that vast knowledge, I knew *one thing* that he did not. One small microcosm of information that made the difference between life and death.

Knowledge, I'd learned, always requires responsibility.

According to the law of the land, I could be judged on two counts: First, for what I knew. Second, for what I *should have known*.

In a court of law, a pathologist might not be held accountable for failing to recognize that little known heart pattern. But as an experienced coronary care nurse, I *should* know it.

It's been more than twenty years since that long winter night. As far as I know, all the players of the drama that unfolded are still alive. When I think of those events, I can't help but believe that someday we as believers will be held accountable by God for what we know and what we should have known through His Word and Spirit.

Clearly, none of us are responsible for everyone. We can't know everything, understand everything, or fix everything. But sometimes I look at the critically wounded world around us and wonder who might have seen the signs and intervened in the lives of the young men who brought death and mayhem to Columbine High School. What friend or neighbor might have recognized the darkness in Timothy McVeigh's tortured soul before he ignited the blast that brought down the Murrah Building in Oklahoma City?

Those of us willing to minister *a healing touch* must learn to look at the people around us with a fresh perspective. Instead of rejection they may need unconditional acceptance, the truth spoken in love, a job, a meal, or simply a word of encouragement.

> *I*f you have knowledge, let others light their candle by it.
> —*Thomas Fuller*

Some years ago a woman who lived across town carefully loaded bullets into a gun, climbed into her car and drove to a remote location to kill herself. Possibly as a result of someone's prayers, she made one stop along the way. A friend of mine owned the business where she stopped. He didn't look past her. He didn't look through her. He took the time to really look into her soul. And he gave her one of greatest gifts a person can give. He listened to her—really *listened*—while keeping one ear open to God.

"Offer her a job." It was a gentle nudge from the Lord, the kind of quiet whisper it's easy to ignore. This man heard and extended more than just an hourly wage—he cared. She accepted his kindness and his job. At home that night she unloaded the

gun and put it away. Much later she explained how his caring in that critical moment had saved her life.

We must understand this about the person who crosses our path:

One more injection of rejection could be their fatal dose.

Refuse to give it.

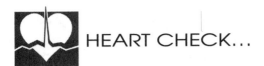 HEART CHECK...

Hopefully you'll never find yourself in a situation like the one that occurred during the dark hours of that long wintry night. But you might find yourself fighting for someone's life through prayer and intercession. You might even have to stand against what everyone else believes is right. In that situation it will be equally important that you know your spiritual rights and responsibilities.

√ **Check your heart by asking these questions:**
  - How would I respond in a similar situation?
  - Are there any of God's laws, written in the Bible, that I know I'm not following? If so, repent and accept responsibility.
  - What has God taught *me* in His Word and through prayer that I'm responsible for?

√ **Get a piece of God's heart.**
  - You can't be all things to all people. Only God has that role. But there are things you can do and people you can touch. Ask God to reveal what part of His heart is yours.

Father, please reveal the things in my heart that have kept me from accepting my responsibility as Your child and joint-heir with Jesus. I admit that You know me better than I know myself and it is only through Your grace that I am changed into the responsible intercessor and healer You have called me to be. Give me Your wisdom to use my responsibility wisely. I ask this in Jesus' name. Amen.

CHAPTER FOUR

I Wanna Volunteer on a Cruise Ship

He went to him and bandaged his wounds, pouring on oil and wine. Then he put the man on his own donkey, took him to an inn and took care of him.
—Luke 10:34

When God called me into nursing in a cow pasture that day, I didn't have any idea what I was signing up for. I talked to a college counselor who listed many varied opportunities for nurses.

"Most people associate nursing with hospitals," she said, "but hospital work is only one of the avenues open to nurses."

She listed other options.

"Many nurses work in doctor's offices," she explained.

Nine to five. Weekends off. I like that.

"Another opportunity is to be a school nurse."

Weekends off. Christmas off. Holidays off. Spring break off. Summers off. It's perfect!

"Some nurses become officers in the military."

I could see the world!

"Even cruise ships have a nurse aboard."

Nursing on a cruise ship? Yeah!

I went to college dreaming of life on a cruise ship. Nothing could have been further from reality.

I didn't know back then that I would spend the better part of the next two decades working for one hospital—many of those years spent in critical care.

I didn't know how exhausting nursing would be. I didn't know how emotionally draining the labor would be. I didn't know I would work ten-day periods, many of them double shifts, not knowing for certain when I would get a day off.

> *T*he world is to be cleansed by somebody, and you are not called of God if you are ashamed to scrub.
>
> —*Henry Ward Beecher*

I didn't know that I would wrestle with the grim reaper for so many years that I learned to smell his presence.

I didn't know that death and I would learn to know one another so well. Or despise one another so much.

I didn't even know there was a spirit of death.

I didn't know anything about spiritual warfare either.

But I learned.

That's why, when my "later years" arrived and I started my second career as a freelance writer, I resigned from nursing with a sigh of relief.

Finally, I could leave death and dying behind me. I had earned the right. Paid my dues. Got out on good behavior.

My life was simple and uncomplicated.

I could do the three things I loved: raise my children, write, and pray.

No more wrestling with death.

Except it didn't exactly work that way. At first, I was amused when the Lord gave me prayer assignments and spoke to me in medical terms.

I figured that was all He had in me to work with.

I figured wrong.

For a while, my prayer responsibility on difficult cases was to assist and support more experienced pray-ers to whom God had given primary responsibility.

Then one day the Lord called me to intercede on behalf of someone with a spiritual heart problem.

Coronary care—my specialty.

"This will be a new experience for you," the Lord said. *"The patient is in critical condition, and you are the Team Leader in charge."*

The Holy Spirit's choice of words caused the hair on the back of my neck to stand at attention. I recalled in vivid detail my first experience as Team Leader in the Critical Care Unit the day of my twenty-first birthday.

I never wanted to repeat that experience. Not in nursing, and not in prayer.

Surely it's just a figure of speech, I thought, consoling myself.

It was not.

Everything in me was tested during that experience.

It was another coming-of-age ordeal; this time in prayer.

The patient and I both survived, but I was beginning to feel anxious about the patterns that I saw being repeated. More and more often, I saw parallels between what I'd experienced in my nursing career and what I was now seeing in intercessory prayer.

Too often the Lord revealed things to me that I did *not* want to know.

I didn't want to know that the wife of a colleague was sitting in her husband's closet with a gun to her head picturing her brains splattered on his best suit. God had triggered me to pray for her, then to phone her. When I called, she described sitting in the closet with a gun to her temple.

Now I knew.

That made me as responsible as I'd been during the resuscitation in X-ray so long ago. I was responsible for what I knew then, and I was responsible for what I knew now.

Once again, I found myself battling with death. Only this time it wasn't in the critical care unit with heart monitors and cardiac stimulants.

It was in the prayer closet.

It was on the phone with the woman contemplating suicide.

Baking a pie for her family.

Driving her to appointments.

Listening.

Did I know her well?

No.

My responsibility was much more serious than just knowing her.

I *knew.*

God never failed any of the people He assigned to me.

Sometimes I did.

In the hours before dawn one Sunday morning, I dreamed of torment and murder.

I watched as a tormented man wearing pressed jeans and a white shirt planned a killing spree. Horrified by the scene unfolding before me, I knew I had to call the police to stop the massacre. Laundry spilled out of the basket and my house was a mess, so I cleaned house, folded clothes, and wrote an article. With all my chores finished, I picked up the phone to dial 911 only to learn that I was too late—two people were already dead. I woke in a cold sweat.

My hands shook while I dressed for church that morning. I knew the man in my dream. He lived a few miles from me. Beyond a doubt, his tormented mind was on the verge of breaking. I cried off my mascara and had to reapply it twice before church.

Looking back, I realize that this was my first double warning dream. Until then, when I knew someone's life was in danger, I always had time to pray it through at my leisure. What I missed was that this dream warned me of two things. First, of impending death. Second, that my own priorities were out of order. The dream warned that I would wait too long to call in the forces of heaven to intervene.

> *E*very calling is great when greatly pursued.
> —*Oliver Wendell Holmes, Jr.*

During church, I couldn't keep my mind on the service. The dream kept creeping into my thoughts like a bad flashback. The gravity of the situation I'd seen in my dream gripped me.

This situation is going to take days or weeks to pray through, I reasoned. I looked at my schedule and saw that I had an article due the next day. In addition, my house was a mess, and the children didn't have any clean underwear.

If I write the article tonight, I thought, *tomorrow I can clean house and do the laundry. Then, on Tuesday, I'll be free to pray this thing through.*

It never occurred to me that I was doing exactly what I'd done in the dream.

On Tuesday morning, with my assignment completed, my house clean, and the laundry done, I promised God, "Today, and the rest of the week, I'll pray for this man as long as it takes."

I walked into the kitchen and glanced at the newspaper lying on the table. The headline hit me like a blow to the solar plexus. For a moment, I couldn't catch my breath.

The man in my dream had murdered his wife and killed himself.

I spent those hours in prayer as I'd promised God, but it wasn't intercessory prayer.

It was a prayer of repentance.

Their blood was on my hands.

I was the watchman God had called to sound the alarm, but I had allowed my "To Do" list to derail me.

"The Lord would have called others to pray too," a friend consoled me.

I agreed. God probably had triggered others to pray. But that didn't relieve me of *my* responsibility. I knew. Just like in critical care nursing, I was responsible. It's that simple.

The more of those similarities I saw, the more uneasy I became. Finally the pattern of battling death every time I stepped into the prayer closet became clear. We were visiting my parents in Wolfforth, Texas, when, laying across the bed in their guest room, I inquired of God.

"Lord," I prayed, "Why do I keep tripping over the dead and dying when I pray?"

Immediately, I recalled my pastor standing in the pulpit a few weeks before saying, "The church is a hospital!"

I'd heard that analogy all my life, but I saw no Scripture to support it.

The Lord reminded me of the story of the Good Samaritan recorded in Luke 10. The Good Samaritan took the man he found by the side of the road and left him in an inn to recover. I'd often heard ministers compare that inn, where the man was nursed and nurtured back to health, to the church. Clearly, one function of the church is to nurse a sick and dying world. We have the life they so desperately need.

In a flash, I realized the parallel. Hospitals, like churches, have administrators and support staff. They have doctors and nurses that dedicate their whole lives to birthing babies—like evangelists in the church. There are pediatric wards where doctors and nurses nurture the children—just like those in the church committed to nurturing baby Christians. They have psychiatric units where staffs spend their lives healing the human soul—the oppressed, depressed, and the possessed.

They have critical care units....

God wanted me to work in a Critical Care Church!

I burst into heart-wrenching sobs. I might not have known what I was signing up for in the cow pasture, but I knew the cost now. I did not want the next twenty years of prayer to be a repeat of the past twenty years of nursing experiences.

"Lord," I sobbed, "if the church is a hospital, I want to volunteer to wear pink and deliver flowers! I'm not doing critical care nursing anymore! I'm *not!*"

"*You agreed to your call long ago,*" the Lord answered patiently.

"I did *not!*" I gasped. "I agreed to nursing for a time. Afterward, when that was finished, I agreed to write."

"I never said your nursing would be finished. I called you into nursing. Period. You were called. The only thing that has changed is the method. First you did critical care nursing in the hospital. Now you do it in prayer. I also told you that in your later years you would write."

I was stunned speechless.

"But I didn't *know* what I know now."

Silence.

"Okay," I said, still weeping, "if the church is a hospital, I want to be reassigned. Lord, I wanna volunteer for a cruise ship."

Silence.

"I'd like to speak to the person in charge of staffing. I'm applying for a transfer."

The Personnel Director had nothing else to say.

It appeared that hospital nursing had been boot camp for the real work ahead.

There were to be no cruise ships for this nurse.

Perhaps you, too, would rather serve on a cruise ship than in an intensive care unit. I'd like to tell you that God's assignments are multiple choice, but they're not. I *can* tell you that the Creator of heaven and earth, the One who hung the sun, moon, and stars in place, is the same One who formed you—wonderfully—in your mother's womb. He has numbered every hair on your head and engraved your name on the palm of His hand.

He knows you better than you know yourself.

> *The place God calls you to is the place where your deep gladness and the world's deep hunger meet.*
> —Frederick Buechner

God may assign you to pray for the president, for children at risk, or to intercede for the course of nations. Whatever He has called you to do—He has equipped you to do.

Cruise ship or war ship—you are programmed to succeed.

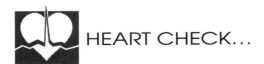 HEART CHECK...

When God calls you to care and prayer in a critical situation, it may not be for a person about to pull the trigger. It may be for a marriage about to implode. It could be on behalf of a teen trapped in drug abuse. It could be for a mother whose unborn child is in trouble, or about an impending road disaster. Accepting your assignments from God is a matter of trust. It means trusting Him to direct you and to equip you for what He's called you to accomplish. If your assignment appears to be impossible, just remember that this is not about you.

It's about Christ *in* you.

√ **Check your spiritual pulse:**

- What assignments are you certain God has given you?
- What is the last thing God told you to do?
- Were you obedient to do it?
- If not, take it to the cross and repent.

Father, help me look at the wounded world around me and be willing to accept Your assignments. Give me clear direction on what You want me to do and how You will equip me to do it. Today I say to You that I'm willing to be willing to answer Your call. I ask this in Jesus' name. Amen.

CHAPTER FIVE

FRIENDSHIP WITH GOD

But I have called you friends,
for all things I have heard of my Father
I have made known to you.
—John 15:15 NKJV

I paid for my food in the crowded lunchroom at a convention I was attending. Balancing my lunch tray, purse, Bible, notebook, and drink, I scanned the area for a place to sit. Two men seated at a tiny table saw my dilemma and made room for me.

We'd been visiting for a few minutes when the conversation turned from the conference to prayer.

"Are you an intercessor?" one of the men asked me.

"Well…" I began, and then paused, "I guess you could say that."

"Wow," he said, shaking his head, "I'm sure glad God never called *me* to *that.*"

"Me, too," the other man added vehemently. "Thank God, it's not my gift."

I felt an immediate, overwhelming urge to cry.

Frankly, the whole argument about whether intercession is a spiritual gift or a call was beyond me. Many times, I'd listened to different biblical scholars whom I respected state their case one way or another. It made my head spin.

I figured that if I were a Bible scholar I would understand. If I were, I might have given those two men the benefit of my opinion. But I'm not. Right or wrong, I wasn't going to argue.

Instead, I finished both lunch and the conversation, then left to find a quiet place to pray.

"Lord," I whispered, "I believe what those men said hurt You. I'm *so* sorry. Who ever heard of a Christian *not* called to pray?"

According to the Bible, now that Jesus is at the right hand of our Father, He ever lives to make intercession. (See Hebrews 7:25.) If the definition of being a Christian is Christ living *in* us, then doesn't it stand to reason that He would be interceding *through* us?

I shook my head to clear it. How could people make something so simple, complicated? Personally, I don't think that God had a senior moment and forgot to list intercessory prayer with the spiritual gifts of wisdom, knowledge, faith, healing, discernment, prophecy, tongues, and interpretations of tongues in 1 Corinthians 12.

Neither do I think He was confused when He listed intercession simply as a type of prayer in 1 Timothy 2:1: *"I urge, then, first of all, that requests, prayers, intercession and thanksgiving be made for everyone—for kings and all those in authority, that we may live peaceful and quiet lives in all godliness and holiness."*

Nor do I see any evidence that God, through Paul's letter to Timothy, was speaking to a called, chosen, or select group of Christians about prayer. As far as I can see, He was talking to *all believers.* The way I read the Bible, believers are to pray at all times with *all types* of prayer.

Why, then, does it seem that most believers in the church spend all their prayer time petitioning God about their own needs, while a few are "called" or "gifted" to intercede?

Personally, I think intercession is simply a choice: A choice to obey or disobey the biblical admonition to pray *"all kinds of prayers"* (Ephesians 6:18).

It's interesting to me that throughout the Bible we see men and women of God standing in the gap for individual lives, for cities, and for nations. Although they were different people living at different times, I noticed that they all had one thing in common.

They were called friends of God.

Abraham interceded before God on behalf of the twin cities of Sodom and Gomorrah. God wouldn't bring judgment on those wicked cities without discussing it with Abraham first.

> *A* friend is a person who goes around saying nice things behind your back.
> —*Anonymous*

Why?

Because they were friends.

Years later, when speaking to Jacob, God said, *"But thou, Israel, art my servant, Jacob whom I have chosen, the seed of Abraham my friend"* (Isaiah 41:8 KJV, emphasis added).

In the New Testament, James 2:23 records that Abraham *"was called the friend of God"* (NKJV).

Hundreds of years later, God chose Moses as an intercessor on behalf of the nation of Israel. According to Exodus 33:11 NKJV, *"The LORD spoke to Moses face to face, as a man speaks to his friend."*

David, the shepherd boy turned king, was a friend of God. The Bible says that David was a man after God's own heart.

I believe that in the midst of every great move of God upon the earth, He has had a friend.

God had friends who spent years praying through His plan. He had friends who boldly preached the Word of God, healed the sick, and raised the dead.

There are a lot of people today who are hungry for the power of God.

I don't believe they are the ones who will experience it.

The ones chosen for the last great harvest are people who are hungry for *God*.

Not power.

There are countless thousands who have studied and become great Bible scholars.

Yet, knowing the Bible is fruitless unless you *know* the One who wrote it.

God does not entrust His power and His glory to great Bible scholars, to expert orators, or great leaders.

He trusts His friends.

Most of God's friends have been unlikely leaders, unlikely scholars, and unlikely speakers.

They were unlearned fishermen like Peter, Andrew, James, and John.

Or plumbers like Smith Wigglesworth, who healed the sick and raised the dead.

Or shoe salesmen like D. L. Moody, another unlikely leader. Moody was never ordained into the ministry, never attended college nor earned a college degree. He was an uneducated man who could hardly spell. But he was a friend of God who presented the gospel to more than one hundred million people over forty years.

They were simple men with a simple goal.

To *know* God.

There are two notable qualities in the friends of God I've known. They are obedient to the written Word of God and obedient to spending time with Him in prayer.

I never set out to be an intercessor. I probably didn't even know the term when my gratitude to Him, and my hunger for Him, drove me to pray.

I didn't know there were different kinds of prayer. But as I spent time waiting before Him, I learned that the Holy Spirit has many different moods. If He felt like singing, we sang. If He felt like weeping, we wept. If He felt like talking, I listened. If I was hurt and wounded, He comforted and healed. If He was grieved over something, He told me, and I spoke His will on earth in prayer.

It was very uncomplicated.

I noticed, though, that in His presence the gifts of the Spirit operated freely. I couldn't help but wonder if that free-flowing stream of gifts of the Spirit—the word of knowledge, the word of wisdom, the gift of faith—was why intercession had been labeled "a gift."

In intercession, as with all types of prayer, the Holy Spirit only took me as far as I asked to go.

Once, years ago, I had been crying out to God in prayer, asking to move to a deeper place in Him. I wanted to know Him more. I was surprised when, in answer, He began waking me during the night to pray.

That wasn't the way I wanted to get to know Him. It certainly wasn't the time.

On one such occasion, I *couldn't* make myself get out of bed at such an hour. Wrestling with my conscience, I finally rolled over and went back to sleep.

A few minutes later, the Lord spoke again.

I believe it was my last opportunity to be used of God in a particular situation.

"What if I tell you this concerns a child?" He asked.

A *child?* I was wide-awake. I pulled myself out of bed and wrapped up in an old quilt. A deep heaviness settled over me as I knelt to pray. I suspected that it was intercession, but I'd never experienced anything quite like it. I soon discovered that my normal place in prayer wasn't deep enough to get the heaviness off me.

A few days later, a friend from Texas phoned to tell me that her ten-year-old son had been admitted to a psychiatric hospital for clinical depression and suicidal tendencies. Once there, he experienced what the doctors called a "total psychotic break."

They predicted that he would never be normal again, and that he probably wouldn't ever be discharged.

I prayed everything I knew to pray for the boy, wondering if perhaps this was the child the Lord had spoken to me about. I suspected that it was, and that the darkness I was experiencing was intercession for him.

But I wasn't sure.

Finally, I decided to do a nursing assessment on my own systems. "Emotions," I asked, "do you have a problem? Is there anything troubling you that would make me feel crazy?"

Nothing.

"Body, are you sick? In pain?"

Nothing.

The darkness I was battling was spiritual, and it wasn't about *me*.

I tried to pray out of my head knowledge, but my head had no idea what was going on. I kept shoving the problem aside because I didn't want to deal with it.

Finally, after about four months, I'd had enough. I needed a breakthrough, and I was going to pray until I got it. I decided to forgo sleep in order to pray until I had victory.

It was the longest night of my life.

I began to pray in the Spirit rather than out of my intellect. I prayed. And prayed. And prayed.

This kind of prayer, I realized, was *work*.

For the first several hours, nothing much happened, except that I felt foolish.

Then sometime after midnight, I grabbed my head in agony. It felt as though strong bird talons were ripping me apart.

I dared not stop praying.

At three o'clock in the morning, I coughed and gasped for air.

Then—it was over.

No heaviness.

No darkness.

No pain.

No feeling crazy.

I went to bed and slept long and sound. The next afternoon, I got a call from my friend in Texas. That morning, she'd received an urgent message from her son's doctor asking her to come in immediately.

"Are you a Christian?" he demanded when she arrived.

"Yes..." she said. "Why?"

"Because something we don't understand has happened to your son. It's as though a light came on inside of him. This morning he woke happy and in his sound mind. Since then, he has gone to every person on the ward telling them about Jesus."

Jesus.

He ever lives to intercede.

Through us.

Jesus suffered and died for everyone in the world to be saved, but if you read the Bible, you'll see that although salvation is offered equally to all, His relationships varied. First, there were the multitudes to which He preached, miraculously feeding the five thousand. Then there were the disciples—twelve men who were given the meaning of the parables. Those twelve were trained to reign. Even so, the Bible portrays a friendship between Jesus, John, and Lazarus that ran deeper than teacher or disciple.

We each begin as one of the multitude and must choose to take one step farther to be a disciple. Only love will woo us as deep and abiding friends.

I believe Jesus is asking us the same question He asked Peter so long ago.

Do you *love* Me?

Friendship is
a single soul
dwelling in two
bodies.
—*Aristotle*

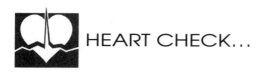 HEART CHECK…

Today the young boy I prayed for is a twenty-eight-year-old Marine. He's not only dangerous to the enemies of this nation; he's also dangerous to the enemy of his soul. When I think of him, I always recall how the Lord taught me to assess the three parts of myself. You don't have to be a nurse to do your own system check. Take a moment right now, and I'll walk you through it.

√ **It's great to get away where it's quiet, but you can do this checkup anywhere:**

- Begin by being still and paying attention to how you feel.

- Focus on your body. Does anything hurt? Isolate any discomfort and make note of it.

- Now focus on your emotions. Is there anything bothering you? Have you got unresolved thoughts or feelings that you haven't dealt with? Make note of them. If there is unforgiveness or bitterness, this would be a great time to repent. If you've got stress rolling around in your mind, take time to pray and cast the care of it onto God. He's more than able to handle the situation.

- This is the part that may be new to you. Now that you've assessed your body and your soul, turn your attention inward. Pay particular attention to the upper abdomen, just below your breastbone. This is roughly the place where your spirit man resides. Do you feel agitated or uneasy there? If so, you definitely need to pray, because this is a spiritual issue.

I've had many situations when circumstances screamed at me that disaster loomed ahead, but this system check gave me great peace. One such time occurred when a relative had a very negative report from her doctor. In the natural, things looked grim, but when I checked my spirit, I found great peace. In time the doctor discovered what my spirit had already told me: She was fine. On another occasion, we got a call that our beloved horse had gotten out of the pasture and strayed onto a busy street where she was hit by a car. My mind was doing cartwheels, but my spirit was at peace. When we arrived on the scene, we found the car had been totaled, but the driver was fine, and Candy had only one scratch.

√ **Now that you know how to do your own system check, get in the habit of doing it often. Learning to rely on the Holy Spirit will make your friendship with God more immediate.**

Father, I have watched You from a safe distance, never close enough that You could change my plans and reorder my world. Like the tide, there have been times when I rushed forward with a kiss only to retreat from Your great love. Call me out of the boat and give me the grace to follow! Call me forth from the stench of my grave and teach me to live again. Let me be Your faithful servant—and friend. I ask this in Jesus' name. Amen.

CHAPTER SIX

PIGGYBACK HEARTS

Greater love hath no man than this, that a man lay
down his life for his friends.
—John 15:13 KJV

I was stunned when I heard the news on December 3, 1967. What happened in Cape Town, South Africa, at Groote Schuur Hospital was nothing short of a medical miracle. I listened to the report on television, then grabbed the nearest newspaper. The headline sent shock waves around the world.

Dr. Christiaan Barnard Performs
World's First Heart Transplant!

Then, like now, heart disease stalked our nation's finest men and women, cutting them down in the prime of their lives. Many people must have read the news like a reprieve from certain death.

Within the next twelve months, one hundred and one heart transplants were performed around the world. I followed the news hungrily, never imagining that more than twenty years later I would have the privilege of meeting Christiaan Barnard when he helped the hospital where I worked develop its own heart transplant program.

Finally, all the questions I'd harbored over the years were answered. I was fascinated to discover that Dr. Barnard hadn't discarded the worn-out heart of his first transplant patient. Although the heart couldn't continue sustaining life, it did function marginally. Dr. Barnard had taken the strong donor's heart and *attached* it to the patient's own heart. The procedure became known as a "Piggyback."

Over the years, Dr. Barnard discovered that there were certain advantages to having *two* hearts—one weak and one strong—sustain a life. Many of the first patients in our transplant program also had the piggyback procedure. I watched in fascination as *two* heartbeats marched across the cardiac monitor screen.

Years later, when I'd left coronary care for a prayer closet, the Lord burdened me for a man in our church. As I began to pray for him, the Lord spoke.

I'm going to perform a heart transplant on him.

My mind flashed back to those patients who'd been given a new life following heart transplants. I smiled. It was so sweet of the Lord to speak to me in medical terms. I imagined myself as the surgical nurse prayerfully assisting the Great Physician.

"Lord," I asked, "whose donor heart will You use?"

"Yours."

I laughed nervously, feeling a bit like Isaac looking about for the sacrificial lamb.

"No, really, Lord...where is the donor heart?"

"It is your heart."

"But Lord, the *donor always dies!*"

"Yes."

"Wait a minute. Let's talk. I don't mind praying for this man, but I certainly don't want to *die* for him!"

"Didn't you ask me to show you a picture of intercession?"

"Yes, but…"

"Intercession is a form of prayer that allows one heart to sustain another. The perfect picture of intercession is piggyback hearts."

"I can see that picture, Lord, but about the donor…"

"What's your problem?"

"My *problem* is *death!* I thought Jesus died on the cross so I wouldn't have to!"

"Why do you think I said, 'Greater love hath no man than this, that a man lay down his life for his friends'?"

"I thought it was a metaphor."

"It seemed more than a metaphor to the Christians who died for rescuing Jews during the Holocaust."

"I see your point."

"Be comforted. I'm not asking for your life-blood."

"What *are* you asking for?"

*"I'm asking that you lay down your **life**—your plans, your time, your agenda—everything dear to your **heart**."*

> The way we view death determines, to a surprising degree, the way we live our lives.
> —Billy Graham

I didn't want to do it.

It might have been different if God had asked me to lay down my life for one of my best friends, but I hardly knew this person.

Worse, his personality was thorny. I couldn't have a conversation with him without getting pricked. I knew it was just his pain showing, but it didn't make me want to sacrifice my life.

Still, it was clearly my assignment. My choices were simple: obey or disobey. Life and death stood in the balance.

Reluctantly, I agreed.

The Lord revealed to me that Satan had planned a mental, emotional, and spiritual assault on this man in order to drive him to suicide. An onslaught he was too wounded to withstand.

Two things happened when I agreed to provide a piggyback heart. First, in a rush of divine grace, I saw the patient through *God's* eyes. Until then, I didn't understand how different each of us must look to God than we appear to the world—or the church.

When I glimpsed who this saint was called to be in God's kingdom, the love of God was shed abroad in my heart for him. (See Romans 5:5.)

Every trace of reluctance fled.

I would willingly die to keep him alive.

The second thing that happened was that all the spiritual, mental, and emotional anguish sent against him—fell on me.

I felt like I was fighting for my life.

I know I was fighting for his.

I still remember the day that God disconnected our piggyback hearts. I had been kneeling beside my sofa praying and thanking God for victory. Afterward, I stood and walked across the room.

Snap.

I knew immediately that something had happened. I went back to the Lord in prayer, and He told me the surgery and healing process had been a success.

I, on the other hand, was exhausted. The year of warfare had taken a heavy toll on my body.

"Why, Lord?" I asked, seeking Him for an answer.

"Do you remember when you and Ken were training for the Dallas White Rock Marathon?"

"Yes, Sir."

"How did you eat then?"

"Well, before long runs we always loaded up on carbohydrates and lots of fluids to sustain us."

"What would have happened if you had eaten normally, as though you weren't running long distances?"

"My body's demand for fuel would have been so great it would have cannibalized its own muscle tissue to get it."

"That's right. And the same thing is true spiritually. Carrying someone in intercession is like running a marathon with another person on your back. You need much more fuel than usual. The Word of God is the bread of life. It is your spiritual fuel."

I was stunned. I hadn't changed the amount of time I spent in the Word during those months. The only thing that increased was the amount of time I spent in prayer. I failed to carbo-load for the race. No *wonder* I was exhausted.

In addition to the lack in my spiritual diet, the Lord had given me a dream with specific instructions for this case. I had followed all His instructions.

Except one.

That one act of disobedience on my part allowed the enemy's forces to regroup and postpone the victory. I had everything I needed for success. I'd been given authority, and the weapons of my warfare were mighty for the pulling down of strongholds.

I had the name of Jesus.

I had access to the blood of Jesus.

I had the gifts of the Spirit.

I had all kinds of prayer.

I had the keys of the kingdom—the power to bind and loose.

I had the Word of God.

I had weapons. I just hadn't practiced using them. I didn't know which weapons were offensive and which were defensive. Even when I did choose a weapon, my spiritual muscles were weak and untrained, and I didn't know how to properly use it. I didn't understand how to wield the authority I'd been given.

For a year, I'd heard the Holy Spirit speak the same warning over and over, but I couldn't figure out what to do about it.

> *There is no exercise better for the heart than reaching down and lifting people up.*
> —John Andrew Holmes

"Satan has you on the defensive. Move to the offensive position."

I didn't even understand those terms in football, much less in prayer. How was I supposed to take the offensive position? What would put Satan on the run?

Finally, I got still enough to hear the answer.

"Do it the same way Jesus did."

Of course! Jesus always dealt with Satan the same way. "It is written..." The spoken Word of God would put Satan on the defense and me in the offensive position! I'd been powerful in praying in the Spirit, but slack in speaking and praying the Word.

"From now on," the Lord said, *"put the Word in first place and praying in the Spirit afterward."*

I opened my Bible, "Thank You, Lord, that according to Luke 21:15, Satan cannot overcome me for God has given me a mouth and wisdom the enemy cannot gainsay nor resist."

I had to admit, praying the Word of God first each day seemed monotonous and legalistic after praying mysteries. But as time passed, I noticed the strangest thing. The fires I'd been trying to stamp out all around me disappeared. The storm still raged, I knew, but it felt like I was in the eye, a place of quiet calm.

The next thing I noticed was that, as I faithfully prayed God's Word, it strengthened my own heart to the point that I stepped up into a new level of spiritual authority.

"Lord," I prayed, months later, "thank You so much for teaching me a new order in my prayer life. My life has changed for the better!"

"Yes," the Lord confirmed, *"it's always best to put Jesus first in your life."*

"What?" I asked.

"Think about it," He said. *"Jesus always reveals the Holy Spirit. The Holy Spirit always reveals the Father. When you pray in that order, the Father will always be revealed in your life."*

Day by day, the Holy Spirit taught me, trained me, and I began to grow in His ways.

On Call in Disneyland

A few years later, Ken, Heather, Lauren, and I arrived at Disneyland—breathless with anticipation. Part of my excitement was seeing my children's eyes light in awe. Mostly, I needed a vacation; a time to put all the intense cases aside and simply have fun.

The first day flew by in a blur of pirate ships, talking animals, and jungle forests. At midnight, after fourteen hours of play, we fell into bed with tired smiles on our faces.

I didn't dream of cartoon characters.

I dreamed one of our friends killed himself.

I saw his wife and three children grief-stricken at his graveside. Then, as if in slow motion, I dreamed the following years and witnessed the devastation that suicide thrust on each member of the family.

The digital clock flashed 2:00 a.m. when I sat up in bed with my heart hammering. I took slow breaths and wiped the perspiration from my face. Finally, I lay back down and stared into the darkened room. Suddenly, the roof of the Disneyland Hotel opened and rolled back like a scroll. I watched the drama of my friend's family continue as though played out on a big screen. I pinched myself...*hard*.

I was awake.

The saga that unfolded before me resembled the classic movie, *It's a Wonderful Life*. Like Jimmy Stewart's character in the movie, our friend had obviously forgotten the gift that God had given him in his own wonderful life.

I was unusually quiet the next morning. Ken, sensitive to my mood, pulled me aside and quizzed me. I mentioned our friend's name. "He's going to commit suicide," I whispered, so the children couldn't hear.

Ken and I had never known anything in this man to suggest that he might be suicidal. But when I told Ken what I'd seen, neither of us doubted it for a moment.

"Forget about Disneyland," Ken said. "We won't do anything else until this is resolved." We put the "Do Not Disturb" sign on the door and started to pray. This time the armor fit nicely. I knew which weapons to use and how to use them.

Satan had spent years setting up this suicide and the following devastation. We destroyed it that morning.

Lighthearted, we went out to play.

We hadn't been home from our vacation long when the wife of the man in my dream dropped by. While taking a walk, I said, "The Lord put your husband on my heart while we were gone. Ken and I prayed for him."

"Really?" she asked, slowing. "Do you remember the date?"

How could I forget? I told her the day we prayed.

"Melanie," she said, stopping in the street to stare at me, "I didn't know it at the time, but that's the day he had chosen *to kill himself!*" She described how, mysteri-

> *T*he heart of a good man is the sanctuary of God in the world.
> —*Madame Suzanne Necker*

ously, that plan had unraveled. Instead of death, he chose life. God orchestrated his wife telling me what happened as a gift for faithfulness, because most times I would never know the rest of the story.

Suicide is the ultimate form of rejecting life.

It's not surprising then that the primary cause of death following a heart transplant is—rejection. Death occurs when the patient's body rejects the heart that is sustaining it.

So what is the prognosis for an intercessory piggyback heart?

With Jehovah-Rapha as the primary physician, the recovery rate is 100 percent.

Unless, of course, a spirit of rejection takes root.

Only, in this case, the patient doesn't reject life.

The intercessor refuses to die.

God asks no man whether he will accept life. That is not the choice. You must accept it. The only choice is how.
—*Henry Ward Beecher*

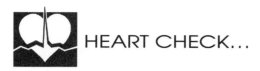 HEART CHECK...

√ **How should you respond if God makes *yours* a piggyback heart?**

- Don't get into pride, this has nothing to do with you.
- Understand that you can't make this happen, but you can refuse the assignment.
- *You* can't save anyone, but God can through you.
- Ask God to protect you from a counterfeit spirit sent from the enemy to wear you down.
- Don't allow the spiritual burden to affect your soul!
- Don't pull the spiritual burden into your soul (mind, will, and emotions) and try to carry it there. Give it to God, and He will carry it for you.
- Spend quiet time listening to the Lord and pray what He puts on your heart.
- Always make sure the Word of God has first place in your life.

Father, I pray that You will teach me about spiritual heart transplants. Help me to always be willing to offer You my heart but protect me from any counterfeit spirit that would try to give me false burdens and responsibility. Keep me from pride and help me understand that this is about You and not about me. Above all, please teach me to pray! I ask this in Jesus' name. Amen.

CHAPTER SEVEN

CORONARY CARE

He heals the brokenhearted
and binds up their wounds.
—Psalm 147:3

*T*he Coronary Care Unit was brim-full of critical patients, but the man in room number seven had kept me running since I started my shift that afternoon. Taking advantage of the current lull, I hurried to set up the evening medication.

"Doctor A! Room seven!" the monitor tech shouted moments later.

Oh Lord, not again.

I bolted to his bedside, where the emergency cart and defibrillator sat waiting. Glancing at his monitor, I saw shark-tooth lines in a fast ventricular tachycardia.

It wasn't conducive to life.

I charged the defibrillator and lifted the paddles. He looked at me with stark terror. "Oh, no..." he whispered. I couldn't tell what scared him most. That I would shock his already burned chest, or that this time, it wouldn't help. He was still getting enough blood to his brain to be alert. But not for long. I decided that the anesthetic of unconsciousness would be merciful. Holding the paddles carefully behind me, I talked to him, soothing him, until he didn't feel a thing.

Clinically, he was dead.

"Clear! Everyone clear?" I shouted to the others gathered around. The electrical charge jolted his large body off the bed by inches. I watched the monitor as his unruly heart straightened up and marched across the screen in perfect order. Moments later, he blinked and spoke.

After the night nurse relieved me, I sat down and counted. If I hadn't been there, and seen the rhythm strips posted, I never would have believed how many times one man could be defibrillated and live. It must be some kind of record.

Yet the man lived to tell about it. A couple of weeks later, he was discharged. For years, he and his wife sent us cards telling of the grandchildren he'd seen added to the family and his travels.

Life.

Sometimes, I realized, the only thing that stands between life and death is a jaw-grinding tenacity that won't give up.

I thought of him again twenty years later when I read the results of my own twenty-four-hour heart rhythm. I diagnosed the arrhythmia that had worsened dramatically over the past few months simply by taking my own pulse.

It wasn't ventricular tachycardia.

But it wasn't good.

No wonder I've been short of breath, I thought, scanning the rhythm strip. The arrhythmia had occurred more than *twelve hundred* times in twenty-four hours! If something didn't change, *I* would end up admitted to the Coronary Care Unit.

Why?

I'd never experienced the kind of fear that gripped me when my heart went wild, flopping like a fish in a boat. Every time I tried to pray, fear gobbled my faith. I needed help. "Lord," I prayed, "I need help! Please call an intercessor to pray for me!"

I refused to tell her anything the first three times she called. It never occurred to me that *she* was the answer to my prayers. I just thought she was weird. I didn't even *know* her, although she was a member of my church. Frankly, I didn't understand anything she said. She talked about pains in her body, "physical words." And the bowels of her compassion being released for me. Didn't I have enough problems of my own? I told her nothing, thanked her politely, and hung up the phone.

I had just walked in the door after reading the results of my twenty-four-hour rhythm strips when the phone rang. It was *her*.

"Look," she said, "I've got to have some relief. I've been suffering physical symptoms in my body for weeks. Each time I ask the Lord about it, He says it's intercession for you. Please, if you won't do it for yourself, do it for me. I'll take off work this afternoon if you'll just let my sister and me come pray for you."

She's my intercessor!?

After seeing my cardiac pattern, I was highly motivated for prayer. "Of course," I told her hastily, giving her directions to my house.

When Deborah and her sister, Jessica, arrived, I started outlining my condition as though I were giving report at shift change. Deborah held up her hand. "Don't tell me anything!" she ordered.

"God called you on my case, but you don't want to hear about it?" I asked.

79

"If I know what's going on," she explained patiently, "I might think I know how to pray about it. That wouldn't help. Besides, what you have to say or I have to say isn't important. The only way to get to the root of your problem is to hear what the Holy Spirit has to say."

"Oh..."

They prayed for a while, asking God for direction. Suddenly, Deborah put her hand on her head. "My head hurts right here," she announced, looking at me with large eyes as though she'd said something significant.

"I have Tylenol®," I said, standing to get it.

"No," Deborah interrupted. "It means that we'll find the root of your problem through a memory."

They watched me expectantly.

"What are you remembering?"

My mind was a blank check.

A while later, they asked me again.

Zip.

"I'm going to lay my hand on your head and pray," Deborah explained. "God will bring the memory up to you."

She'd no sooner done that than it all came back to me. One of those experiences you'd rather not remember. It washed over me like waves—brokenhearted, suffocating agony, humiliation, anger, unforgiveness, hatred...

Hatred?

It boiled up like bile in my throat.

I'd never known it was there growing in the garden of my heart.

I learned a valuable lesson that day.

Repentance is the great deliverer.

Forgiveness the great healer.

Two hours after they'd arrived, Deborah and Jessica left. For the first time in three months, I went to bed and slept soundly. No sitting up gasping for air. No knocking in my chest like an engine out of tune. No fear twisting my mind like a rag.

None of those things happened the next day, either.

Or the next.

By the time my doctor saw my rhythm strip on Monday, the cardiac arrhythmia that had worsened continually for more than a year was gone.

"Lord," I cried, thinking of all those years of heart monitors, needles, and defibrillators, "I like Your way better!"

"The coronary care units," He said, *"are full of brokenhearted people."*

> *T*he heart has eyes that the brain knows nothing about.
> —Charles Parkhurst

Ten years passed while my heart beat out a strong, steady rhythm. Meanwhile, I studied under the Holy Spirit's school of healing broken hearts.

"Would you like to know the material that has hardened his spiritual arteries?" the Lord asked me one day about a recent prayer assignment.

I stopped in my tracks.

Spiritual arteries have plaque? I wondered in awe. I stood still, thinking. Our physical bodies require blood to sustain life. Our spiritual hearts require the blood of Jesus for life. Life is in the blood in both realms—physical and spiritual. I thought about the Lord's words. *"Would you like to know the material that has hardened his spiritual arteries?"*

The word "material" riveted me. In the human heart, that material is called plaque. Some of it is soft and pliable. It can be pressed easily against the artery wall by angioplasty. Other plaque is hard and brittle. I realized that there must be different kinds of spiritual material that block the completed work of Jesus' blood in a heart.

What could they be?

"Yes, Lord," I finally answered, "You have my undivided attention. What is blocking this man's spiritual arteries?"

"Despair."

Despair! Deadly despair. I knelt to pray everything I knew to pray against despair. *"No!"* the Holy Spirit ordered.

"No?" I asked. "You don't want me to pray?"

"I want you to sing to his heart."

So, He's in a singing mood today.

The words welled up in my heart before I ever uttered the first note. "God will make a way where there seems to be no way..." The power of God wrapped itself around those words like the beam of a laser light shining into a man's heart.

That was all. A song and a dance before the throne of God.

The only thing the Lord enjoys more than touching a human heart, I realized, is doing it in such a way that it shakes up religious thinking. I knew for this situation, I'd done all that the Lord required of me. There was no sense in my trying to pray with many words out of my understanding. There were too many things I *didn't* understand.

I couldn't help wondering what other "materials" were used to block spiritual blood flow. A few weeks later, the Lord revealed another one to me.

"Would you like to know what material forms the hardest, most brittle hearts?" the Lord asked. *"Those hearts that are hopeless apart from a miracle?"*

I tried to imagine what kind of sin would harden a heart that seriously. Was it idolatry? Murder? And who were those people?

"Yes, Lord," I answered, "I want to know what causes the hardest of hearts, but first will you show me a scriptural picture of them so I'll know what kind of people you're talking about?"

"Look up Jeremiah 17:1."

I turned to the passage and read, *"Judah's sin is engraved with an iron tool, inscribed with a flint point, on the tablets of their hearts."*

I'd seen human, fleshly hearts many times over the years, but I couldn't imagine any heart so hard it could be engraved with an iron tool. Even more shocking, the people with the hardest hearts mentioned in Jeremiah weren't the Philistine army. They weren't the inhabitants of Sodom and Gomorrah. God was talking about the tribe of Judah! God's chosen people! The very descendants of Abraham and Isaac! They were in covenant with God. He had delivered them out of the hand of their enemy! He had healed their sick! These people knew more about God than anyone else on the face of the earth at that time.

"Now look in the New Testament at Matthew 13:15."

I turned to Matthew and read, *"For this people's heart has become calloused."*

I stared at the words of that verse for a long time. Here, the Lord was talking about the Pharisees. Again, they were God's chosen people. They were descendants of Abraham. They not only knew more about God than any people on earth, they knew His law. They didn't just quote their favorite Scripture promises.

They could quote whole *books* of the Torah. Yet, the Word of God itself condemned them. Somehow, they had God's Word engraved in their minds, but not in their hearts.

"Lord," I asked, "what material caused the hearts of Judah and the hearts of the Pharisees to become hard?"

"Satisfaction."

I gasped. *Satisfaction* is the deadliest form of spiritual heart disease?

I began to see the picture. God brought the Israelites out of Egypt with great signs and wonders. But Israel was satisfied with Egypt.

God gave them a land flowing with milk and honey, but they didn't want to fight giants. They were satisfied on the other side of Jordan.

The Creator of the universe made Himself their King. They were satisfied with a human one.

I thought about the Sadducees and the Pharisees living in Jesus' day. They were satisfied with their religious customs, traditions, and rules.

God wouldn't fit in their box.

So they nailed Him to a tree.

What about us? I wondered.

Most Christians in the world today know more about the Bible than anyone in the history of mankind. Many of us began memorizing Scripture verses before we could spell our names. We have Bibles in every room of our homes. We have Bibles in every translation. We have Bible commentaries. We have the Bible on our computers. We hear the Word of God on television and on tapes.

We are good people, raising good children, and serving a good God.

We are *satisfied* with that. Even though a million lifetimes wouldn't allow us time to know all the facets of God we could explore through prayer, we were satisfied with the thimbleful that we have experienced.

In a flash of understanding, I knew that those who step forward for intensive caring will never be satisfied.

Until the yokes of bondage are destroyed.

Until the brokenhearted are healed.

Until the blind can see.

Until the lame can walk.

Until those who are bound have been released from their satanic bondage.

Until the last trumpet blows.

Today, God is using coronary care units in hospitals around the world to save as many lives as possible. They will continue to do that until the church gets dissatisfied watching a weeping, wounded world.

*G*od can do
wonders with a
broken heart if
you give Him all
the pieces.
—Victor Alfsen

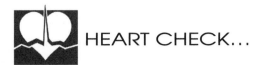 HEART CHECK...

√ **Tips on sustaining a healthy heart.**

- Check your heart daily for unforgivenenss—and *choose* to forgive.
- Lift your brokenheartedness to God and ask Him to heal it.
- Never get too spiritually satisfied.

Father, I ask that You heal the brokenness in my heart and deliver me from a crushed spirit. Your Word says that hope deferred makes a heart sick, so I ask You to keep my hope and joy alive and well. Deliver me from a broken and crushed spirit and heal me spirit, soul, and body. Make me an instrument of Your peace. I ask this in Jesus' name. Amen.

CHAPTER EIGHT

ORDER IS NOT
A FOUR-LETTER WORD

Let all things be done decently and in order.
—1 Corinthians 14:40 NKJV

*A*ttention! Code Blue! Room 840! Attention! Code Blue! Room 840! Please refrain from use of the elevators until further notice.*" The telephone operator's voice quivered as she announced the emergency over the public address system.

I dropped the chart in my hands, pitched the narcotics keys to the nurse setting up evening medication, and ran. Inside the staircase, I heard the steps of other team members echoing as they ran up to the eighth floor.

I was breathing hard by the time I opened the door from the stairwell to the eighth floor. Grateful for the respite from stairs, I ran the rest of the way to room 840, where a patient had suddenly died. As part of the Code Blue Team, I was required to respond to the resuscitation in progress. The instant I crossed the threshold into the room, I started counting the people who'd already arrived. In an emergency situation, with nurses and doctors arriving from all over the hospital, it was impossible to function as a member of the team without first knowing your order.

87

By counting the number of people in the room, I knew my job was to start an IV and administer drugs. I grabbed a tourniquet and dropped beside the bed to find a vein in the lifeless arm. As soon as the needle was in place and the fluids dripping, I gave the first dose of sodium bicarbonate.

An observer would have thought that the people who arrived in room 840 that day had worked together for years because we functioned like different arms on the same body. That couldn't have been farther from the truth. We had never had this exact mix of people in this exact order. In an emergency, you don't have time to ask, "What do you need me to do?" "Who is doing what?"

The reason we didn't need to stop and ask questions was because we knew the drill. Countless times when I was training for the Code Blue Team, I'd heard the announcement and run to the designated room. Instead of a dead patient, I'd been met by the team's medical director with a stop watch in his hand and a dummy in the bed.

"You're the second to arrive!" he barked like a drill sergeant. *"What do you do? Show me!"*

"You're third to arrive! What do you do? Show me!"

"You're fourth to arrive! What do you do? Show me!"

Knees shaking, I had scrambled to remember the responsibility assigned to my order. We held the mock resuscitation as though it were real. *"The monitor shows ventricular fibrillation! What do you do now?"*

The person handling the defibrillator had better remember to shout, *"All Clear?"* before shocking the dummy. We were scored and rated on every move we made and every word we spoke—or didn't speak. Afterward, he reviewed everything we'd done right and everything we'd done wrong.

My heart rate didn't usually settle down to normal until long after I'd returned to the relative safety of my own unit. As frightening as those drills were, they were also the reason we could run to a resuscitation anywhere in the hospital and, without question, do what needed to be done. It became second nature to count.

1...2...3...I'm fourth!

1...2...I'm third!

1...I'm second!

In nursing, order establishes both responsibility and authority. It is impossible to fulfill your responsibility without knowing your order.

Order wasn't just an issue when facing a crisis. Every day, during each shift, we found our order. Some days, I was the Team Leader in charge, and the older, more experienced nurses were in staff positions. Other days, I was a staff nurse with a different order and authority.

My order in the Coronary Care Unit gave me a great deal of responsibility. Yet, if I walked onto the seventh floor, I had no administrative authority. That was someone else's role. Still, if I saw a problem, there were spheres of order and authority that I could operate within.

However, if I responded to a code blue on the seventh floor, I functioned in two realms of authority. First, I found and operated in my team order—derived numerically by when I arrived on the scene. In terms of decision-making during the resuscitation, I walked in great authority. If a cardiologist or internist were present, as a coronary care nurse I ranked second in command. If any other doctor was present, I had the final say if a question arose about how to proceed. Those decisions had been ordered by the hospital medical staff.

Order wasn't something set in stone and never changing. To walk in order you had to learn to flow, much like a marching band on a field seems fluid as it takes different shapes.

Order in a hospital is so logical that I was surprised to discover that many Christians think of order in the church as a four-letter word. Order is no more or less than what its name implies. It brings *order* out of chaos.

Besides, God offers great blessings to those who will find and stay in their proper order. A good example of that is Elijah and Elisha. God called Elisha to be in order behind Elijah. Showing great wisdom, Elisha never stepped out of that place. God blessed him with a double portion of the anointing on Elijah.

Joshua was an aide to Moses during all those years in the wilderness, and according to the Bible, there were times when Moses, having met with God, went back to his tent. But Joshua stayed in the presence of God. When others murmured, complained, and rebelled against Moses' authority, Joshua was never counted among their number. After forty years in the wilderness, Moses only got to see the Promised Land from a distance. Joshua had the privilege of leading Israel into their inheritance.

David, the shepherd boy, was an armor bearer for Jonathan, King Saul's son. Once again, David never stepped out of his order with Jonathan, and he never tried to step around Saul, even after the Lord had removed His hand from the king. Yet, God anointed David to be king over Israel and promised to establish his throne forever.

Christians who try to promote themselves and step out of their God-given order have forgotten that the kingdom of God works opposite from the world's system. In the world, success comes from climbing over other people in the scramble to be at the top. In God's kingdom, the last will always be first.

If you look at the earth, or the universe, it's easy to see that our God is the God of order. The Bible is full of its symbolism. Mark 4:28 says, *"All by itself the soil produces grain—first the stalk, then the head, then the full kernel in the head."*

He brought order to the sun and the stars as recorded in Genesis 1:5, *"God called the light 'day,' and the darkness he called 'night.' And there was evening, and there was morning—the first day."*

He ordered the building of the ark. He ordered the Red Sea to part. He ordered the building of the temple. He ordered the morning and evening sacrifices.

> *Order is heaven's first law.*
> *—Alexander Pope*

He's about to bring new order to the church in these last days.

If ever the body of Christ needed order from chaos, it is now.

He is restoring to the church the fear of the Lord.

He is restoring an awe of His Word.

He is restoring the prophet to warn the church of coming events.

He is restoring the apostle to rally the armies of God for the greatest harvest of souls ever known.

He is restoring the intercessory watchmen to watch and pray over the world.

There is a new order coming to the church. Not organization—order. The anointing of God has nearly been organized out of the church, but God is making a clean sweep. Those of us who dare to rise to the call of God must learn to flow in *His order.*

He is mobilizing the church for a great awakening.

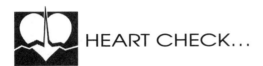 HEART CHECK...

Don't get locked into traditions of men that have no place in the next move of God. Recognize that the body of Christ is made up of believers from every denomination. No one group has all the answers. This is no time to be a sheep lagging alone behind the flock. Find your assigned place in the church, and don't leave your post.

√ Ways to stay in order:

- Ask God where He has assigned you and get planted in that church.
- Never go AWOL (Absent Without Leave). God isn't schizophrenic. He isn't confused about where you should be. Find your place, and don't leave without clear direction.
- Submit to spiritual, governmental, vocational, and familial authority.
- Once you're *under* authority, you will *have* authority.

Father, I repent of any ways that I've been out of Your order. Plant me firmly where You have called me to serve, and help me respond to those in authority over me as though I were responding to You. I ask that You not only bring order to your church, but that You bring order to my life and my home. I ask this in Jesus' name. Amen.

CHAPTER NINE

THE AWAKENING

Wake up, O sleeper, rise from the dead, and Christ
will shine on you.
—Ephesians 5:14

I shined a bright light into the blank eyes of an eighteen-year-old head injury patient. His pupils reacted minimally in response to the glare. It was one of the few signs of life in the once robust young man. His strapping six-foot frame lay flaccid; his arms and feet rotated inward in a position typical of head trauma. He didn't respond to deep, painful stimuli. He didn't flinch when I restarted his intravenous fluids. I dropped medication into his eyes and taped them shut to keep them lubricated.

He couldn't even blink.

The ointment seeped from the corners of his eyes like tears. I knew they *weren't* tears, but those glistening drops on his eyelashes made him look as miserable as I felt.

I hated taking care of head injuries.

Usually, neurological cases went to another floor of the critical care tower. My primary responsibility was cardiac patients. I loved them. You had to fight for their lives, but when they stabilized, they moved to a step-down unit within a few days. And a whole new batch of critical cardiac patients filled the beds.

Occasionally, like in the case of this young head injury, the medical-surgical ICU would overflow into our unit. The thing I disliked was seeing them *lifeless* for so long. Day after day and week after week passed with no change. A month passed, then another. After four months, excitement rippled through the staff.

He blinked!

A blink of an eye was enough to keep some nurses going for weeks.

I was more impatient.

Still, I knew that there was nothing more exciting than an awakening. The day it happened was worth all the waiting. The moment when lifeless eyes came alive. When limp, cold fingers wrapped around my hand and squeezed. That first spoken word.

The moment of recognition when a son speaks his mother's name. When a husband calls for his wife. An awakening is second only to Lazarus stepping out of his tomb wrapped in grave cloth. Or when Jesus, risen from the dead, walked through walls and visited His friends.

An awakening is exhilarating. For the months leading up to the event, the patient may have been present physically, but he was absent in every other way. It is as though they are reborn.

So why didn't I long to work the neurological ICU?

Because I knew what to expect on both sides of that blessed event. On the front side, months of waiting and wondering if they would ever awaken. After the event, there were months and months of hard labor. In those months, the newly awakened patient sometimes had to relearn years of knowledge.

Like how to talk. How to feed himself. He had to relearn how to walk and how to throw a ball. He had to relearn what a hammer was, and how to control his bowels and bladder.

Those developmental stages are fun when a toddler holds your finger and takes his first tentative steps. It isn't quite the same experience when you are trying to steady someone who outweighs you by a hundred pounds.

That's not to say it isn't rewarding. Every milestone is significant. But it is a slow process that requires infinite patience, especially on the part of the family. They bear the brunt of the burden.

It still felt like a miracle a year later when my young patient sauntered back into the unit to say hello. Tan and muscular, there was no resemblance to the boy who'd lain still for so long.

Then, it was all worth the wait.

I looked into those laughing eyes and thought it hadn't been long at all. A brief moment in time. Head injuries have always been the best and the worst for me.

The waiting is excruciating.

The awakening is exhilarating.

One is certainly worth the other.

Years after I'd witnessed my last awakening in the intensive care unit, I had reason to think long and hard about head injuries again. I was attending a conference in Dallas, Texas, when it happened. The conference speaker seemed to fade into the background. In the Spirit, I saw a woman, dirty and disheveled, slouched in a chair. She appeared to be in a drunken stupor. Two men approached and mocked her. They opened her blouse and lifted her skirts to stare, laughing at her nakedness.

"Lord," I whispered, tears streaming down my face, "who is she?"

"She represents the church in America," the Lord replied, *"but she isn't drunk as you suppose. Don't get haughty because you're awake. You have only awakened in response to someone's prayers."*

That woman represented *us*?

Is that what we looked like in the Spirit? What I saw had been described in the book of Revelation. I read the words that God spoke to the church of Laodicia:

> *For you say, I am rich; I have prospered and grown wealthy, and I am in need of nothing: and you do not realize and understand that you are wretched, pitiable, poor, blind, and naked. Therefore I counsel you to purchase from Me gold refined and tested by fire, that you may be [truly] wealthy, and white clothes to clothe you and to keep the shame of your nudity from being seen,* **and salve to put on your eyes, that you may see.**
>
> (Revelation 3:17–18 AMP, emphasis added)

We desperately need that salve put on our eyes. I realized in a flash of revelation that the world is unconscious to Jesus because the church is asleep to His manifest presence. The world will never awake until the church awakes.

I heard a friend teach on living in the manifest presence of God. "The first thing most of us were taught about the presence of God," she said, "is that you can't live there."

At that moment, I realized that we'd been lulled to sleep by a lie.

Of *course* we could live there. The first Adam had lived in His presence. That's why the second Adam—Jesus—went to the cross. He purchased the right for us to live in His presence, eternally. Like the unwise virgin, we fell asleep waiting for His return.

All the while, He'd been here for us through the Holy Spirit. He'd been waiting for us to awaken and live in His presence.

I *had been* that woman in my vision, I realized. Someone had nursed me in prayer and put spiritual salve in my eyes until I'd opened them and recognized Him—Jesus.

How long and patiently I had been nursed. I had been milk-fed at first, until I could chew spiritual food. I learned to walk leaning on others until the day that I could stand alone. I had been taught, loved, and discipled. I began looking at the world around me with new eyes.

Now my heart's cry was to awaken to His presence daily.

A few weeks later, I picked up a copy of *Charisma* magazine. *"A Special Report,"* the cover read. *"Are We Headed Toward Revival?"* It was the subtitle that riveted my attention. *"Many Christian leaders believe we are on the verge of global spiritual awakening. Here's what you can do to prepare for it."*

A worldwide awakening? Those people will need one-on-one care!

I thought about my favorite book, *Rees Howells: Intercessor*. In one chapter, Rees recalled the great revival that swept through Wales in 1904. He said, "But the real problem arose as the revival proceeded and thousands were added to the churches. There were more children born than there were nurses to tend them."[1]

God will do His part, I thought, *but are we prepared to do ours?*

That evening a friend phoned. "My family rented an old movie," she said. "It's called *The Awakening*. Have you seen it?"

I remembered the movie well. It was based on an actual medical case of a doctor who worked with a group of neurological patients who'd been in a coma-like condition for years. They were trapped inside their own minds, unable to escape, unable even to speak.

The doctor, who was dissatisfied with their plight in life, experimented with dosages of a drug developed for Parkinson's disease. Miraculously, each of the patients awakened from their comatose states. Those awakenings had been as exhilarating as any I'd ever imagined.

But the effects were only temporary. Eventually, they each returned to their previous state. I shuddered, trying not to imagine a spiritual awakening where, due to lack of care, those who'd been brought back to life fell back again into darkness.

"Sure," I answered my friend, "Robin Williams played the doctor."

"That's the one," she agreed.

"What about it?"

"The Lord told me it's a picture of a spiritual awakening."

Awakening. I'd given anything if God had given her a picture of people who stayed awake. I knew it was a warning. I couldn't speak.

"The thing that occurred to me," she continued, "is that if there is an awakening, we'll need a lot of nurses."

I sighed. Intensive prayer and intensive care. Milk-fed. Spoon-fed. Taught, loved, discipled. Each and every one. Until all the risk of remission is gone.

It's just a movie, I thought. *People don't waken to the presence of God only to nod off again.* Even as the thought formed, I knew it wasn't true. The parable of the sower and the seed in Matthew 13:18–23 taught that the cares of this world could choke out even His presence. Those cares, I realized, washed over us like rhythmic waves, hypnotic, lulling us to sleep.

The example my friend gave was one I had lived year after year growing up in the church. Each and every summer, I attended an awakening called church camp. Those glorious days were filled with an electric thrill of God's presence.

We sang. We wept. We prayed. We awoke.

Then, back in our home churches, we stood in the pulpits and testified that we were forever changed. We would *never* be the same again.

The adults patted our backs and smiled knowingly. They knew. They'd seen it year after year. They had experienced their own youth camp awakenings. Then, like the people in the movie, like us, they'd fallen back unconscious of God's presence.

I stopped with my children at a convenience store recently. The music from a car that pulled alongside us shook my windows. "Look, Mom," my daughter said as they piled out of the car. They were a sight to behold. They wore black leather jackets with chains wrapped symbolically around their waists. Their hair varied in hue from green to purple. They sported snakes tattooed on their arms, rings in their noses, lips, eyebrows, and ears.

I waited behind them in the checkout line, positioning myself to look into their eyes when they turned to leave. Their blank stares looked hauntingly familiar. I had the sudden, inexplicable urge to drop ointment in their eyes and tape them shut.

"Why do they dress that way?" my daughter asked when we were back in the car. I turned to look into her bright, beautiful eyes. Eyes that were awake and alert to both worlds around them.

"It's a head injury," I muttered. My daughter looked at me closely. "Head trauma makes you do strange things," I said. "They need intensive care. Really, they need intensive prayer. Let's pray for them now."

After we prayed, I felt an old stirring of excitement. I wanted to be there. To see the light in their eyes. To help them take those first teetering steps. I would willingly spoon-feed them. I'd do anything to see them awaken to God's presence.

They will be fearless and full of faith.

They will never be ashamed of the gospel.

They will shake the world.

The sinners are asleep in the darkness, while the church is asleep in the light.
—Keith Green

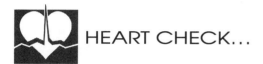 HEART CHECK…

√ **Pray and ask God for an awakening if you have any of these symptoms:**

- Spiritual apathy
- Lack of joy
- Tendencies to control and manipulate
- Anxiety and panic
- Spiritual boredom
- Greed
- Seared consciousness to sin
- Addictions

Father, I pray that You would forgive me and cleanse me of any of the symptoms of spiritual sleepiness. Awaken me to Your Spirit! Teach me to learn to live in Your presence! Prepare me to pray and offer a helping hand to others as they awaken from deep sleep. Help me to nurse them until they are living in Your presence—fearless and full of faith. I ask this in Jesus' name. Amen.

CHAPTER TEN

THE RACE

Therefore, since we are surrounded by such a great cloud of witnesses, let us throw off everything that hinders and the sin that so easily entangles, and let us run with perseverance the race marked out for us.
—Hebrews 12:1

On the first day of my new job at our hospital-based fitness center, I wore enough white to blind an Eskimo. My new position was to supervise the cardiac rehab patients whose physicians had referred them to our facility. The transition from intensive care to cardiac rehab was not an easy one for me. The first time I took a group of cardiac patients to exercise on an outdoor track, I carried a portable defibrillator under my arm. Within minutes, the wind had tinged my blazing white uniform dirt red.

I couldn't help notice that Kathy, a physical therapist, was doubled over laughing at me. It was hard to act indignant when she intercepted the nurse's cap that blew off my head and into a nearby field. "It's time to lighten up," Kathy said, trying to stifle her laughter as she relieved me of the defibrillator and sat it on a nearby bench.

"But, what if…"

"If we need it," Kathy reassured me, "it will be right here."

I eyed her T-shirt, shorts, and running shoes with envy as sweat soaked my thick white hose. So much for turning a fitness center into an intensive care unit. Nobody needed a defibrillator that day. Or the next. As hard as it was to accept, these patients weren't critical any longer.

I retired my white uniforms, opting instead for running shoes and loose, comfortable clothing. I reported arrhythmias, inappropriate blood pressure responses, and helped the physicians monitor side effects of the patients' medication. I taught classes on heart disease and helped the patients develop both work and vocational goals. Then we set about achieving them.

Gone were the adrenaline rushes of intensive care nursing.

Gone were the thrills of fighting for someone's life.

Lord, did I make a mistake by taking this job?

I didn't hear any response from God.

Until I met a patient I'll call Bill.

Bill, a fairly young man with a wife and two sons, had just been discharged from the hospital following a massive heart attack. He was still suffering severe chest pain. I reviewed the films of his heart at work, especially watching the movement of the left ventricle—the heart's primary pump. I felt a lump in my throat. Only a small portion of the inferior wall moved at all.

His heart was inoperable. His prognosis was grim—perhaps six months to live. His cardiologist referred him to us for emotional support.

Death had been hard enough to deal with during those first critical days following a cardiac event. Having survived that only to face a lingering demise was a dismal prospect for Bill to endure, and for me to watch.

After our usual ten weeks of exercise sessions, Bill still experienced severe chest pain brought on by very little exertion. Our entire team of nurses, physical therapists, exercise physiologists, occupational therapists, dietitians, and social workers met to discuss Bill's case.

After reviewing all the data, we agreed that his situation didn't look promising.

"With so little of his left ventricle still functioning," Kathy explained, "his most pressing problem will be avoiding congestive heart failure."

"That's right," the dietitian agreed, "although he isn't overweight, I suggest that he lose down to his lean body mass and maintain a low fat and low sodium diet."

"He's young to face a lifetime of severe diet restrictions," the social worker added. "What will motivate Bill to stick with it?"

"The truth," Kathy interjected. "Let's sit down with him and show him the films of his heart in motion. Let's explain the risk of congestive heart failure and give him not only hope, but a plan."

"That sounds great," another member added, "but we've got a man with severe angina on exertion. Nothing we've done so far has helped. Is there anything to be done about that?"

I couldn't think of a thing.

"I suggest four more weeks of rehab," Kathy said. "We'll work one-on-one with him to push back his angina."

"Push back his angina?" I asked. I'd never heard of such a thing. "In the CCU, we treat angina by pushing the patient back to bed."

"In the CCU, you were working with a coronary event in progress," Kathy reminded me. "Pushing back angina is a result of the training effect. The exercise will train his skeletal muscles to extract more oxygen from the blood stream as he works, thus reducing the workload on his heart."

Kathy outlined her suggested plan. "We'll teach Bill how to differentiate between four distinct levels of angina," she said. "With constant cardiac monitoring, and one minute blood pressures, we'll exercise him through level one angina. At the onset of level two angina, we'll treat him with nitroglycerin and continue his exercise. We'll stop at the onset of level three."

Although I understood the physiological basis for her recommendations, I also knew that it was subject to human error. What if Bill missed his cues for the different levels of chest pain? What if, instead of walking him through levels one and two, we walked him through levels three and four? Level four was a polite way of saying the patient was experiencing a full-blown heart attack.

It wasn't Kathy's understanding of human physiology that prompted me to support her plan. It was my growing understanding of Kathy. At only thirty years of age, she held the dubious honor of being the world's longest survivor of stage four Hodgkin's disease. Stage four was the most advanced stage of the cancer. At age eighteen, Kathy had been admitted to the National Institute of Health to take a new experimental drug. One by one, other patients in other stages of the disease died.

Obviously, Kathy lived, although her disease was the most advanced.

"The medicine was a breakthrough," she had admitted when I quizzed her. "But there was one other thing that wasn't factored into the study."

"What was it?" I asked.

Kathy had sipped a cup of hot coffee and gazed out the window, reluctant to tell me.

"What...?" I asked again.

Kathy sighed and turned to look at me. "I don't know if you can understand this," she said, "but I never saw myself dead. Not once. Not ever. Not when I was too sick to lift my head. Not when my hair fell out. Not when the radiation fried my pericardium. Not when surgeons removed the pericardial sac around my heart. Not when I suffered from radiation-induced heart failure. I never saw myself dead. It wasn't an option I ever entertained."

I thought about Bill. Everyone, it seemed, was looking at the data and seeing him dead. Everyone except Kathy. That's why level four angina didn't scare her. She'd faced and conquered her own fourth stage. If anyone could guide him through the maze of cardiac land mines that faced him, Kathy could do it.

"All right," I said, "let's do it."

We didn't pull any punches with Bill. We showed him his films and talked straight about what they meant. The dietitian laid out his eating plan. Kathy explained his exercise plan.

Since the day Bill had been told that his heart was inoperable, our plan was the only shred of hope he'd been offered. He grabbed it like a lifeline.

The only person who experienced palpitations when Bill walked on the treadmill was *me*. Exercising a man with chest pain went against everything in me.

But this man wasn't in the coronary care unit.

Then, he had fought for his life, now he was fighting to live.

There was, I realized, a difference.

107

I checked Bill's blood pressure and noticed the sheen of perspiration that covered his face. "Angina?" I asked. He nodded.

"What level?"

"Two," he said, rubbing his chest.

I gave him a nitroglycerin tablet and rechecked his blood pressure.

At first, he developed chest pain at an exercise heart rate of 90...then 94...98...100. By the end of the four weeks, Bill could exercise up to a heart rate of 114 without pain!

He graduated from cardiac rehab and became a member of the fitness center. A few weeks later he returned to work. Soon afterward, he asked to meet with Kathy and me.

"I never get chest pain anymore unless I use my arms," he explained. "I can walk anywhere I need to go, but pulling open a heavy file drawer triggers pain. I used to enjoy hunting, but now holding a rifle triggers chest pain too."

"Training is specific to the muscles used," Kathy explained. "We can train the muscles in your arms the same way we trained your legs to work more efficiently."

Bill continued his regular exercise program and added sessions pedaling an arm ergometer. Soon, he was pulling open file drawers and hunting without pain.

Bill was faithful to both his diet and exercise plan. The six months that he was expected to live passed without incident. A year later, he was still doing well.

His face became a familiar sight several evenings a week during his second year. And a third. Eventually, he had no symptoms up to a heart rate of 150.

Finally, Bill had a new problem.

His muscles were so adept at extracting oxygen that he couldn't walk fast enough or walk up a steep enough incline to raise his heart rate. Without an increase in the intensity of his workout, he would lose his training effect.

"There's only one thing to do," Kathy said, her blue eyes sparkling. "We're going to have to let him run."

Kathy and I presented ourselves to Bill's cardiologist. "You want to do *what?*" he asked. After we presented all our data, he reluctantly agreed.

For the next few weeks and months Kathy and Bill were a common sight on the outdoor track. She started him at no more than a shuffle, then worked up to a slow jog. In helping Bill, Kathy was battling her own radiation-induced heart problems. But run she did.

Six years after Bill first walked through the doors of our fitness center, he asked us to help him meet another life goal. "Sure, Bill," we said, "what now?"

"I want to enter the Tulsa Run," he said.

I was stunned. *A 9.3 mile race?*

Of course not! I wanted to scream. *It's been six years! You're not just some patient who passes through the double door and then leaves! You're a part of us now. You're our friend. It's not that you can't risk it. We can't risk it!*

"I don't care about my time," he hastened to add, sensing my dismay. "I just want to go the distance and finish the course. I need to do this. You could help me train."

Kathy loved nothing better than a challenge. She was lit up like a Christmas tree. "We've got until October," she said. "I say he does it. And I'll run it with him."

I wasn't sure who worked harder to prepare—Kathy or Bill.

Race day dawned overcast and dreary. The rain started before breakfast and continued all day. In spite of the weather, thousands of runners bolted when the race began. Everyone, that is, except Bill and Kathy. They started out at a slow jog to conserve their strength.

Most of the fitness center staff, and many of the members, showed up for the momentous occasion. We stood in the drizzling cold and watched runners cross the finish line. In time, the race was over, the finish line removed, and the spectators left.

All except a small group of us who strained for a glimpse of Kathy and Bill. Finally, we saw them shuffling up the last long hill. Forming a human chain where the finish line had been, we screamed and cheered as they closed the distance.

Instead of loosing our hands when they reached us, we wrapped ourselves around them in a group hug. In the middle of the circle, Bill looked up and wept.

"I did it!" he screamed.

I held my face against his soggy shirt and felt the rain mix with my tears.

No defibrillator can give a charge like this.

I've thought about that day many times in the passing years. Bill has become a symbol to me of an important lesson.

It's not enough to save lives.

Our job isn't done until they run their race.

And win.

*F*ar better it is to dare mighty things,
to win glorious triumphs, even
though checkered by failure, than
to take rank with those poor spirits
who neither enjoy much nor suffer
much, because they live in the
great twilight that knows not
victory nor defeat.

—*Theodore Roosevelt*

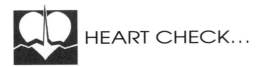 HEART CHECK...

√ **Signs and symptoms of a winning heart:**

- Are you reaching for the impossible or settling for second-best?
- What dreams, desires, or plans have you given up?
- Are you willing to let God resurrect them?

Father, forgive me for settling for less than Your best for me. You are the ultimate Winner, and I am made in Your image. Please resurrect those things You called me to accomplish that I've laid down. Help me to breathe on them the mighty wind of my words. Help me understand that I can always win if I don't give up. I ask this in Jesus' name. Amen.

CHAPTER ELEVEN

FINISH THE COURSE

The race is not to the swift.
—Ecclesiastes 9:11

The Tulsa Run—October 1985

It was a perfect fall morning when I stepped out of my hotel with a race number pinned to my T-shirt. The Tulsa Run—one of the most prestigious races in the country—drew runners far and wide to its 15K course in downtown Tulsa. That morning, thousands of runners gathered to warm up at the starting line. I glimpsed famous world-class runners, knowing full well that once the gun blast started the race, I wouldn't see them again until the awards ceremony.

Like thousands of others, I had no illusions about winning. I hadn't entered the race with even the hope of placing in my age category. I was a slow, steady runner who, when trained, could find my steady-state oxygen level and last for a comfortable five miles. I did not, it seemed, have a fast-twitch muscle fiber in my body. Runners like me had only one goal in mind that morning: Finish the course.

I thought back to the three different years I'd trained for this run. The first time, in 1983, my husband, Ken, and I had run half the Dallas White Rock Marathon—approximately 13 miles—and I knew I could handle Tulsa's 9.6 mile course. Two days before the Tulsa race, I'd doubled over in gut-wrenching pain. I was admitted to the hospital with a partial bowel obstruction. I lay in a hospital bed with an IV dripping in my vein and watched the race results on television.

Next year, I vowed. *I'll run the race.*

The following year, our daughter, Heather, was born, marking the end of those long leisurely runs that Ken and I enjoyed before work. With his busy law practice, my hectic job, and a new baby, we snatched time to run when we could.

Still, by October of 1984, I knew I'd trained enough to finish the course. I was at a department head luncheon the day before the race when suddenly, inexplicably, I gasped in pain and pushed my plate away. That afternoon I was slapped back into the hospital with a partial bowel obstruction.

I was too sick to care about the race results.

A few days later, every symptom left my body as quickly as they'd arrived. Within a week, I was running again. *I'll enter the Tulsa Run in 1985*, I promised myself. *And I'll finish the course.*

The year between Tulsa Run 1984 and Tulsa Run 1985 flashed by in a blur of activity, including the addition of our second child, Lauren. Ken and I discovered that we didn't know the meaning of the word *exhausted* until we had babies twelve months and two weeks apart.

Now, as I stretched my muscles to warm up for the 1985 Tulsa Run, Ken was at home with two children under the age of two. In atypical fashion, he was boycotting the race because he so disapproved of my running. I sighed.

He had reason.

The day before, in a coincidence almost too bizarre to believe, it had all started again. By now I recognized the pain that made me break out in a cold sweat.

Not again.

I'd had a few brief episodes of bowel obstruction over the years, but nothing like I experienced each October before race day.

"The fallopian tube we saved during the surgery to remove your ovarian cyst had been stretched ten inches long," my doctor explained. "The tube is open and functioning, but it's so long that it occasionally acts as a tether obstructing your bowel.

"So far, the obstructions have been partial and temporary. But someday it will block your bowel totally. You won't have much time to get to surgery. *Never* travel outside the country— it's too dangerous."

There were lots of things the doctors said I should *never* do. As far as Ken was concerned I should *never* have driven to Tulsa to run this race.

As soon as the symptoms began, I'd stopped eating and drinking. Now, I was about to run a race dehydrated. Worse, I was running a low-grade fever.

"*Why?*" Ken had asked incredulously the night before when I packed an overnight bag for the trip to Tulsa.

"I just *have* to," I tried to explain.

"But *why* do you have to?" he asked, his voice an octave higher than usual.

"I don't know." And I didn't. I understood the risk. It didn't make any sense to run, yet I couldn't remember ever feeling so *compelled* to do something illogical.

"What could possibly make you feel compelled?" Ken asked, trying hard to understand.

"I...don't know."

Maybe it was because I was sick of being sick.

Maybe because I *hated* being sidelined.

I felt like the devil was taunting me. He'd drawn a line in the sand and dared me to cross it. To me, that line had come to symbolize the finish line of the 1985 Tulsa Run. Something deep inside me screamed, *Finish the course!*

But how could I make Ken understand when I didn't understand myself? I nodded wearily when he said he wouldn't go to the race with me. I'd probably make the same decision if I were in his place.

At breakfast race day morning, I stared at the menu for a long time. I hadn't eaten anything in twenty-four hours, and my physical symptoms hadn't increased. But, every runner knows you need carbohydrates and fluids to sustain you during a long run.

If I ate, the pain might sideline me again.

If I didn't, I might not have the strength to finish my course.

Throwing caution to the wind, I ate half a bowl of oatmeal.

I had chills when I neared the starting line. Perhaps the chills were from the fever, but more likely the thrill of the race. Bright colored balloons floated in the breeze. Grandstands had been assembled for the awards ceremony. Huge digital clocks marked time. I'd never experienced anything like the corporate excitement of thousands of people gathered to run—for no other reason than the God-given ability to do it.

I was toward the middle of the throng when the gun fired. The blast jolted me with adrenaline, and if I hadn't been so packed into the crowd, I'd probably have run too fast and exhausted myself in the first mile.

As it was, the sheer numbers wouldn't let me move too fast. At the half-mile marker, the crowd began to thin out as faster runners sped ahead and the slower runners found their pace.

It was the most perfect morning I'd ever seen. I felt alive in every cell of my body. The air was crisp and cool with the promise of an Indian summer day. Time didn't matter to me as I set a comfortable pace, enjoying every moment of the race I'd almost missed.

Just before I reached the first mile marker, one of my coworkers appeared next to me, matching his stride with mine. Richard, also a registered nurse, was working with the pulmonary rehab patients. Richard was a strong, fast runner—not a plodder like me. While he didn't have a chance to win the race, he could easily place in his age category. Like most of us, he was racing against himself and his own best time.

I assumed he'd started at the back of the pack and was making his way up to the faster runners. *He'll watch for an opening in the crowd and move up soon*, I thought.

But he didn't.

"Richard," I said after a while, "you're missing your openings. Move on up and run at your pace."

"I think I'll just stay and run with you," he said.

That's when I *knew*. He must have gotten a call from my husband.

Ken wanted a nurse running beside me!

I shook my head and sighed. I hated to see Richard throw his race, but there was no way I could run his pace. "Please, Richard," I begged, "run your race."

"I am," he assured me. "I'm comfortable running with you. By the way...how're you feeling?"

117

Hundreds of people lined the streets cheering, encouraging, and urging us on. Volunteers passed cups of water into our hands as we passed.

"You're almost to the three mile marker!" they yelled.

"You're looking good!"

"You're gonna *make it!*"

"You can do it!" perfect strangers screamed as we passed.

"Great job!" faster runners said as they passed us. Everyone, it seemed, had a word of encouragement. The crowd mentality seemed to be, *Some will be fast and some will be last, but we're all in this together!*

As we neared the five-mile marker, I knew I was about to pass my comfort zone. Most days, I could run five miles comfortably, but dehydration and fever were making me work harder than usual. The party would be over for me at five miles. The next four-plus miles would be sheer force of will.

I can do it, I told myself, imagining the rush I'd get as I neared the finish line with its cheering crowds, band, and flying confetti. I grinned. I'd never wanted anything in my life like I wanted to finish the course—and cross that line.

I shifted mental gears as I passed the five-mile marker. *Conserve strength...stay steady...keep putting one foot in front of the other.*

Suddenly a tall man a few lengths ahead of me fell. He didn't fall forward, but sideways. His six-foot frame lay squarely across my path.

I'd seen enough death to know he was dead before he hit the ground.

The situation was clear: I could stop my race and resuscitate him. Or I could step over his body and finish my course.

"*No!*" I wanted to scream. "This is *my* race! This is *my* course! This time I get to finish my race. I don't want to be a nurse right now. Why did he have to die *here?* Why *now?* Why *me?*"

Everything in me wanted to step over him and never look back.

But I couldn't.

Richard and I broke stride and dropped beside him at the same moment. I felt for a pulse. "He's dead," I said, confirming what we already knew.

For a brief moment, as hundreds of feet ran past us, Richard and I looked at one another and shook our heads at the irony. In a race of thousands, this man dropped dead in front of not one, but two, intensive care nurses.

"You'll have to breathe for him," I said, drinking in huge gulps of air. "I'm too short of breath."

Richard tilted the man's head, cleared his airway and positioned his mouth over the man's mouth. I put the heels of my hands over his sternum as I'd done thousands of times before, forcing the blood out of his heart into his vital organs.

"One one-thousand," I said, counting each contraction.

"Two one-thousand."

"Three one-thousand."

"Four one-thousand."

"Five one-thousand." *Swoosh.* Richard forced air into his lungs.

"One one-thousand."

"Two one-thousand."

"Three one-thousand."

"Four one-thousand."

"Five one-thousand." *Swoosh.*

"One one-thousand…"

The pounding steps as runners parted and passed us kept cadence with our rhythm. The race faded. The spectators faded. I hardly noticed the passage of time.

Two other runners stopped to help. Doctors. We hardly had to think, we knew the drill so well. An ambulance arrived with equipment. We put paddles on his chest...

Finally, the cardiac monitor showed a rhythm. His chest rose and fell. The gray skin around his mouth turned pink. Onto a stretcher. Into the ambulance.

"Stand on the back of the ambulance and hold tight," the driver offered. "I'll slow down as we pass your hotel so you can jump off."

I looked around. The sun had moved far across the sky. There were no runners in sight. No spectators. No water stations. The mile markers were gone. The race long since finished.

I wanted to cry, but I was too tired.

I climbed onto the back of the ambulance, finding a bar to hold. Both doctors hopped aboard. Richard stood in the street squinting against the afternoon sun, an unreadable expression on his face.

"Hurry, Richard!" I said as the driver climbed into the cab.

Instead, he silently, gravely held out his hand to me.

"What?" I asked, puzzled.

"Get off," he said, his eyes piercing mine. "Finish your course."

"Richard, the race is *over!*"

He didn't move, his hand still extended.

The ambulance engine roared to life, its lights flashing.

I jumped off as it screamed away.

I looked around. We were 4.6 miles from the finish line. Except there *wasn't* a finish line now. I was tired, shaking from exertion. My muscles were cold and sore. There was no excitement. No cheers of encouragement. Just rolling hills that looked like mountains.

Silently, we started to run.

I lost track of time. We'd been running two miles when my muscles began to cramp. I slowed to a crawl.

Richard slowed beside me. I could hear his words with each footstep.

Fin-ish-the-cou-rse…Fin-ish-the-cou-rse… That's all that mattered now. Just finish. One step and another.

We were about a mile from the finish when I saw Ken—one baby on his back, another in his arms. *He came after all.*

"What *happened?*" he asked. Richard told him. I couldn't spare the breath to talk.

"Keep going," he urged. "You've only got another mile."

It felt like it was all uphill.

The street was lined with confetti like leftovers from a New Year's Eve party. The stands had been dismantled. A few teens with leather jackets and mohawks loitered on the corner—staring at us as we passed.

The time clock was gone.

Richard and I came in dead last. So far behind the slowest runner that, officially, we never finished.

But as I topped that hill and passed the place where the finish line had been, I finally understood. The race that the apostle Paul had challenged the church to run wasn't a flat track.

It was an obstacle course.

A course lined with the dead and dying.

A course littered with divine appointments.

On an obstacle course, the competitors aren't judged merely by how fast they reach the awards ceremony, but by how they handle the obstacles along their path.

The early church wanted to step over the bodies, too. That's why they asked Jesus, "Who *is* our neighbor?" (See Luke 10:29.) *Surely not the stranger who slows us on the way to the cheering crowds.*

Jesus answered them with the story of the Good Samaritan.

> *B*ut he that
> endureth to the end
> shall be saved.
> —Matthew 10:22 KJV

He was just a man who saw the unlovely lying beside the road. Many others passed him by. Even a rabbi or two. Hurrying to the synagogues for their awards ceremony? But the Good Samaritan diverted his course. His awards ceremony is yet to come. He'll stand before the Judge of all judges—before the greatest court of the universe—and receive his award.

Then he'll cast his crown where it belongs.

At Jesus' feet.

Today, the Holy Spirit has slowed His pace to match your stride. I warn you though, He isn't leading you to the accolades of the awards ceremony. For the church, it comes in the next age.

For now, He is leading you to the critically wounded on *your* course. He never promised that the course would be easy. But you have His Word that He will never leave you.

Right now, He is extending His hand. He's pleading.

"Finish the course."

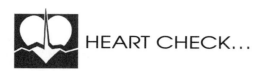 HEART CHECK...

√ **How to discern divine appointments:**

- Recognize that obstacles on your path may be divine appointments.
- Ask God to give you compassion for the spiritually wounded and dying.
- Pray for those who seem to slow your pace.
- Let the Lord teach you to love the unlovely.

Heavenly Father, thank You so much for slowing Your pace to match mine. Thank You for running my race with me and leading me to the divine appointments on my course. Teach me to discern those that You have put in my path for a purpose and grant me the compassion to love the unlovely. Thank You for loving me in my most unlovely state. Help me to love You more. I ask this in Jesus' name. Amen.

CHAPTER TWELVE

SIDELINED

*Restore to me the joy of your salvation and grant me
a willing spirit, to sustain me.*
—Psalm 51:12

An orderly from the psychiatric unit brought her to us. She seemed out of place in the middle of fitness members, tan and strong, who were training for a marathon. Cardiac patients walked briskly on treadmills and pedaled stationary bicycles, yelling to one another over the sound of the equipment and teasing the staff.

She stood like a corpse where the orderly had left her. Her skin was pasty white, her thin body motionless, and her eyes bleak. She appeared to have checked out of life the way most people check out of a hotel. It was as though she turned in her key and said, "I'm out of here."

I'd never seen anyone outside the hospital look so…dead. Sure, she still had a pulse and blood pressure. Her heart still pumped, and somehow she must have been breathing, although her breath was so slight that I couldn't detect movement.

She reminded me of hundreds of people I'd seen like her at St. Louis State Hospital, where I'd taken my psychiatric training. Some devastation had left their bodies intact, but destroyed their souls. I tried talking to her, but she wouldn't speak. Kathy arrived, took her by the hand, and led her outside.

Slipping out the door, she cringed as if in mortal pain. The darkness of her soul couldn't stand the light. She shaded her eyes from the sun as Kathy led her to the track. Still holding her hand, Kathy started to run, pulling her along. While she didn't have the will to live, neither did she have the strength to resist. Still, the sunlight, the wind, the movement was so full of life that she shuddered at the onslaught.

The goal of any rehabilitation program is to stabilize the patient's condition as quickly as possible and get them back into the race of life. The process is key to the recovery of anyone following a life-threatening event.

Psychiatrists at the hospital where I worked grasped the importance of this step of recovery. Several of them began ordering their severely depressed patients to be released from the psychiatric unit an hour a day—into our care at the fitness center.

These pale, withdrawn, apathetic people hardly had the emotional energy to walk across the room. Most were too depressed to carry on a conversation. Left alone, they would stand or sit in one position, lost in the abyss of their minds. It didn't do any good to tell them to exercise.

They couldn't do it.

One of us would take them by the hand and walk them outdoors to the track. Staying close by their side, we set the pace. They followed, feeling the sun on their faces, the wind in their hair, and muscles they hadn't used in months or years.

Always, at the end of a run, their cheeks were flushed and their eyes seemed a bit brighter. They carried themselves more erect and held their heads higher. They wore their victory like a sign.

I accomplished something today!

Day after day, we saw the despair that darkened their countenance lighten.

Doctors say that exercise releases endorphins—a morphine-like substance—into the brain. God is a genius. He built all sorts of life-saving devices into our bodies. He did it, I'm convinced, because the cry of His heart is that every person who has been sidelined get back into the race.

There are many things that sideline people: sin, sickness, despair, satisfaction, hatred, unforgiveness, offenses, pride, haughtiness…the list seems endless.

Satan is the one who sidelines.

God is the One who restores.

Why then, in this last great race that will culminate the end of this age, does the church have the reputation for killing its walking wounded?

Too often, we don't know what to do with them.

Those who commit to intensive caring won't kill—they'll heal. I didn't know about things like that when, in my twenties, one of my best high school friends, I'll call her Jenny, lost her way. Like those psychiatric patients, she just checked out one day. Said, *"I'm out of here!"* And killed herself. When she died, I lost my way.

As I look around the church today, some of our youth, like my friend, are wandering around lost. You can see the questions hidden behind blank, guarded looks.

When does the race of faith begin for me? When I'm old enough to vote? When I'm old enough to drink? When I'm married? When I'm thirty, like Jesus was? When I've memorized a certain number of Scriptures? Would you mind telling me…what's the magic number?

Some days, I want to grab them up and look in their blank eyes. "Those things aren't qualifiers," I would love to say. "They're works. And works stink just as badly when emanating from a child as from an adult.

"There is only one qualifier," I would explain, "His name is Jesus! He is qualified to run this race. Oh, and I have more good news, there is no Junior Jesus. The Holy Spirit is full-grown—in you. The moment you gave yourself to Him, He drew a line in the dirt and fired the gun that started your race!"

I attended a prophetic conference where the speaker called all the youth forward.

Tell them they're qualified! my heart urged. *Get them into the race.*

I shouldn't have worried.

That was God's heart-cry too.

"This is the starting line!" the speaker declared, marking a spot at the front of the room. "The place where you start running your race! When I give the signal, *Run!*"

They ran.

I wept.

Some bolted like bulls from a chute. Others held back, timid and unsure. Some, embarrassed, started and stopped. Some wandered off course. Each time that happened, the speaker took them by the hand and led them back into the race, running with them around that huge auditorium. Shoulder to shoulder, until they found their pace.

Those young giant-slayers will not lose their way.

My friend didn't have that woman in her life. Someone to wipe the tears, tend the hurts, heal the broken heart, and tell her she was qualified. Someone to take her by the hand and lead her back on track. To run with her, shoulder to shoulder, until she found her stride.

Someone to help her up when she fell. To forgive when forgiveness was in order. To help wipe away the filth and grime of shame and condemnation.

Satan's ploy worked perfectly. Jenny died, and I let bitterness sideline me. For five long, miserable years, I never darkened the door of a church.

My friend's death prompted me to study the subject carefully, and as a coronary care nurse, I had ample opportunity to see people die. I noticed that people fell into two groups. The first group, by far the largest, were those people who didn't die well. They struggled, fought, and seemed tormented. Even after death, they didn't look peaceful.

The other group seemed to step over into another place as though they'd just stepped outside. No torment for them. Their bodies may have been ravaged, but their souls were at peace.

It didn't take a rocket scientist to discover the difference, though it wasn't what I wanted to hear. The peaceful group knew Jesus.

Soon after, a new patient was admitted to my care. One that would mark a change in my life more than any patient I'd ever known. *Should the Judge die*, I reasoned within days of his becoming my patient, *his passing would be peaceful*. This man had been brilliant. He had not only written significant rulings and opinions, but prestigious law books as well. His wife and grown children hovered around his bedside, talking to him as though he understood.

Sadly, he'd had so many blood clots fire off to his brain that there didn't seem to be anybody home. The damage, doctors feared, was irreversible.

Although he couldn't feed himself, didn't know where he was, and couldn't remember anything, his face broke into a wreath of smiles when anyone spoke to him. Under the most trying of circumstances, he was always kind and gentle.

Other patients I'd encountered had been very civilized while in control of their faculties. But when that veneer of control was gone—well, it wasn't pretty.

As days rolled into weeks while I nursed the Judge, I found myself going home from work each evening feeling sad and empty. He had an inner spark of joy that no blood clot could remove. I felt cheated that I'd never known him when he was lucid.

God, it seemed to me, had died with Jenny. Except when I was around the Judge. For some unknown reason, God seemed real there—close enough to touch.

His family, especially his wife, believed that God would perform a miracle and heal him. The pastor of their church came by daily to pray.

I stood with my arm around his wife the day the doctor gave her the news. A series of EEGs had confirmed that the Judge, for all practical purposes, was brain-dead.

I had lost all objectivity where this patient was concerned. I didn't want to be the comforter. I wished, for once, that I could throw myself into the collective arms of the family and be comforted. So strong was my reaction to the news that I had to fight for control of my emotions. I heard the conversation in bits and pieces.

"We'll transfer him to a nursing home," the doctor said.

"No...I'm taking him home."

"You can't take care of him. He can't even feed himself."

"God will heal him."

"Be reasonable...."

She wouldn't, for one second, be reasonable, and I knew it. I adored that unreasonable love she held for her husband.

"Melanie," she said, wiping her eyes a while later, "our pastor is here, and we're going to pray. Please, dear, won't you join us?"

What could I say? The truth? That I'd rather stick needles under my fingernails?

Reluctantly, I joined the circle while they prayed. Afterward, his wife patted my shoulder. "He'll be fine once we get him home," she said with the assurance of a brain surgeon.

"You *can't* take care of him," I cautioned.

"I know," she admitted. "That's what I want to talk to you about. I want *you* to do it."

> *T*hings do not change; we change.
> —*Henry David Thoreau*

"Me?" I asked, shocked. "You know I have a full-time job here at the hospital."

"Yes, but only in the evenings. Couldn't you spend the day with us? I could take care of the night and evening shift."

"It's too hard," I argued. "You can't do it."

"Well, what if I hired nurses for the evening and night shifts? Would you come then?"

Of course I would.

The Judge's grandchildren made a huge "WELCOME HOME!" sign that stretched across the front of their farmhouse. Meanwhile, he was lifted like a baby onto the stretcher for the ambulance ride home. When it pulled to a stop in front of their house, he lifted his head and looked out the window.

Something happened in that split-second. Something with God's fingerprints all over it. "I'm home," he said with a huge smile, "and look what those children have done!"

When the finger of God touched the Judge that day, it wasn't a partial work. He remembered everything from the names of all his grandchildren to the most intricate details of law.

The only thing he *didn't* remember was the three months he spent in the hospital. While the Judge and I now had a future, we didn't have a past.

"I'm sorry," he said when I arrived to take care of him, "I don't believe we've met."

He never did remember me from the hospital, but the memories we made when he first walked across the living room were monumental. Another milestone was the first time I helped him to a chair in the yard. By the time he was able to walk around the Olympic-size swimming pool, I knew he wouldn't need me much longer.

Three months after his discharge from the hospital, the Judge went back to the bench. I often remember those days talking and walking beside him in the soft morning sun. I know God must have smiled at the sight we made—wise old gentleman and cynical young nurse. It was a match made in heaven.

I rehabilitated his body.

He rehabilitated my faith.

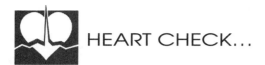 HEART CHECK…

I don't know of a single person who has lived such a sheltered life that they haven't been sidelined, at least temporarily. There are probably as many ways to get sidelined as there are people with stories to tell. Some of the more common ways this happens is through physical sickness, an emotional blow, abuse, injury, failure, a grave disappointment, discouragement, or despair.

√ **Does your faith need rehabilitation? If you have any of the following symptoms, pray and forgive everyone involved in the situation. Then ask God to heal your heart.**
- Bitterness
- Feeling like a victim instead of a victor
- Resentment
- Hopelessness
- Despair

√ **How have you been sidelined?**
- Physically?
- Emotionally?
- Spiritually?
- In fulfilling your dreams?

Father, I pray that You would heal me, deliver me, and get me back into the race. Show me my starting line and run alongside me shoulder to shoulder. Rehabilitate my faith, and help me to be an instrument of healing for those who have been sidelined around me. I pray this in Jesus' name. Amen.

CHAPTER THIRTEEN

WINSTON WEARS SHOES

In the same way, let your light shine before men,
that they may see your good deeds and
praise your Father in heaven.
—Matthew 5:16

I paused over the instruments I was sterilizing to glance out past the large tropical shutters on the window. Lush green trees heavy with fruit dotted the landscape in Montego Bay, Jamaica. I'd traveled here with a team of twenty-nine medical and dental volunteers to staff a temporary free clinic set up in a neighborhood church.

I'd never felt so out of place and discouraged in my life. It wasn't just the heat, or the fact that I was a coronary care nurse trying to function as a dental assistant. It was the need. Crowds gathered around the church at four in the morning, and hundreds still stood in the heat each evening when our exhausted team staggered out of the building. Nothing could have prepared me for that river of human misery.

Sweat ran from my forehead down the goggles I wore and dripped onto the mask covering my face. An oscillating fan blew the paper drapes I'd fastened over the patient's blouse but did little to relieve the heat. The door that separated our tiny work area from the waiting room opened. Judy stood in the doorway, and I glimpsed William outside on the balcony. Theirs were jobs I didn't envy. Judy manned the waiting room, talking, consoling, and trying to fill out necessary papers. William handled the throng that crowded up the narrow stairs outside.

"I'm sorry to interrupt," Judy apologized, "but William says there's a man outside who's in agony."

Don, the dentist, stood and rotated his weary shoulders. "Okay," he said. "I've given this lady more Xylocaine, and we need to let it take effect. Grab a mirror and probe, Melanie, and let's go look at this guy."

Outside, William introduced us to Winston, a Rastafarian. Long dreadlocks fell down his back from under a stocking cap. Out of habit, I did a brief nursing assessment. Large, overweight male. Haggard pain lines across his face. Poor color. Slightly short of breath. Barefoot. Feet: extremely swollen, almost purple.

> *I* believe that life is given us so we may grow in love, and I believe that God is in me as the sun is in the color and fragrance of a flower—the Light in my darkness, the Voice in my silence.
> —*Helen Keller*

Lord, help him, I prayed, *he needs more than we can give him here.*

"Oh...." Don moaned, looking in Winston's mouth. Turning to me, he spoke briefly. "Abscessed. They're all abscessed."

He placed a gentle hand on Winston's shoulder and asked, "How long have you been hurting like this?"

"Long time, Doctor," Winston answered. "Hurt so bad I cannot sleep. You pull them out?"

"Too much infection, Winston," Don said. "I'll give you penicillin, and you come back on Friday."

I pointed mutely at Winston's feet. Winston dismissed my concern with a wave of his hand. "No problem...no problem. Cannot wear shoes. This," he said, pointing to his swollen jaw, "this hurt."

I watched with a sigh as Winston staggered down the rickety stairs.

No problem—a common theme in Jamaica. It seemed to me that all Jamaicans *had* were problems. The contrast between beach-front opulence and the poverty a few blocks away left me bewildered. I'd been confident that our highly trained group would solve a multitude of problems in Jamaica. How wrong I'd been.

During our thirty-minute lunch break each day, nurses and doctors from the medical clinic described their patients. One ten-year-old boy had been too weak to attend school for two years. His problem had been easy to diagnose. Diabetes. He'd never seen a doctor before. His parents simply couldn't afford it.

I was no stranger to poverty. I'd volunteered for a free clinic in Oklahoma City for ten years. There, we'd see everyone who waited if we worked until late at night. But I'd never experienced such a crush of people with overwhelming needs as I saw on this island paradise.

Each passing day brought an increased frenzy to the waiting crowd. Women described spending the last of their grocery money on bus fare to bring their children from distant villages to the clinic.

Each night I tossed in the heat and tried to dismiss the faces of those who still waited. I thought of Winston and wondered if the penicillin would work in time. I wondered if he too tossed in the heat, kept awake by pain. I couldn't help but wonder if his swollen feet suggested congestive heart failure. Mostly, I wondered if anything we were doing was enough. *Your people are hurting, Lord,* I prayed, falling into a fitful sleep.

> *I* cannot say "our" if religion has no room for others and their needs.
>
> —*Anonymous*

Friday morning—the last day of the clinic—dawned bright and clear. In unspoken agreement, our team gulped down breakfast. No time for an extra cup of coffee. We had to press. Doctors, nurses, lab technicians, counselors—all trying to see as many patients as possible.

Don looked at me anxiously when Winston arrived. Judy ushered him past the waiting crowd into the examining room. Adjusting the light, Don and I both leaned forward to see if the penicillin had worked. Yes, the infection was better. If only we had four more days to treat him with antibiotics. "I can't leave him like this," Don murmured.

"I agree," I answered, pulling up several syringes of Xylocaine. An hour later, Winston stumbled out of the dental office on swollen bare feet. Gauze pads were pressed into the cavities where abscessed teeth had rested. My heart lurched as he lumbered down the stairs. *What if...?* I worried, but the next patient was waiting.

By evening, tempers flared as team members struggled to see just one more patient. "Time to close up shop," came our orders.

Don and I ducked our heads, trying to pass through the frantic crowd.

"Doctor, I hurt..." "Please..." Hands reached out to plead and tug for help.

During the bus ride back to our quarters that night, I felt drained. I listened numbly as Monty, our mission director, reported the results of our efforts. We'd treated twelve hundred people in four days. Not bad. I knew the folks back in our home churches would be pleased.

But they hadn't seen the despair on the faces of hundreds of people we couldn't treat. Our team hadn't made a dent in the needs of the Jamaican people. The team hadn't made a dent in the needs of the people in Haiti two years earlier. I thought of Africa, India, our own poverty-stricken people at home. We were a small group up against a world of need. It seemed pointless.

That night, I slipped out of the meeting room where plans were being discussed for a return trip to Jamaica. I walked down to the bay as the sun set. Suddenly, the lingering rays dipped below the horizon, leaving total darkness. For a moment, it seemed that the darkness of pain and poverty had stamped out all the light. I couldn't tell the ocean from the sky, the city from the village.

In that moment, I remembered what one of our team members had said the night before. *"The lights around the bay come on one by one."*

Just then a single tiny light twinkled across the bay. Then another. Transfixed, I watched dozens, then hundreds, of lights flicker on. Soon the city was bathed in light that danced on the water, cutting through the darkness.

Lord, I wondered, *is that all You expect? Each person shining his light where he can?*

On Sunday, our last day in Jamaica, I stood in church with a whole new perspective. Twenty-nine people shone their light for a time in Jamaica. Two churches in Oklahoma had joined hands with a church in Jamaica to make a larger light. Others would come. Other lights would shine.

"Melanie," someone whispered, "you have a visitor." I looked through the shuttered church window and saw Winston. He was grinning. When I went outside, he handed me fruit, necklaces, and bracelets.

> *There is not enough darkness in all the world to put out the light of even one small candle.*
> *—Robert Alden*

"For you," he said proudly, "for Doctor Don...for William... for Judy." Overwhelmed, I stared at the bounty that represented a fortune to Winston.

"See," he said, moving his jaw around, "no pain. Look," he said, pointing to his feet, "the swelling is gone. Now I wear my shoes." I stared in awe at his shoe-clad feet. *You didn't change the world,* the Lord seemed to say to me, *but you changed Winston's world.* Suddenly, that was more than enough.

The bus began rolling away from Faith Temple Church. Winston jogged alongside, shouting, "Miss...Miss!" he called. "You come back next time? Will you come back?"

Reaching out the window, my small white hand was suddenly enveloped inside his burly black one.

"No problem, Winston," I said.

No problem.

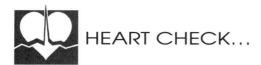 HEART CHECK...

There may be times in your life when you feel as I did facing the darkness and poverty in Jamaica, times when you feel helpless in the face of the overwhelming needs in the world around you.

√ **Check your heart with these simple steps:**

- Make yourself available to God.
- Ask the Lord for both compassion and a glimpse of His heart.
- Where do you think God wants you to shine your light?
- What person or groups of people have needs that tug your heart?
- What ministry or mission could you link up with to help?
- Remember, you can't change the world, but you can change one person's world.

Heavenly Father, I pray that You would infuse me with Your compassion and give me a glimpse of Your heart. Direct my steps and all my ways that I might do Your will on earth. Please light the candle of my life and cause it to shine in the darkness. And Lord, help me to change the whole world...for just one person. I ask this in Jesus' name. Amen.

CHAPTER FOURTEEN

SIGNS AND SYMPTOMS

*This will be a sign to you: You will find a baby
wrapped in cloths and lying in a manger.*
—Luke 2:12

B ack in Jamaica for my fourth trip with the medical
mission team, I used the sleeve of my yellow dispos-
able gown to wipe away the perspiration that dripped
from my forehead to my goggles, blurring my vision. This year, I
worked part of the day in the dental clinic and spent the remain-
der doing evangelism. "Forceps," Don murmured, never looking
up from the patient's mouth where his long fingers worked nim-
bly. I placed the forceps in his gloved hand and turned to pick up
the gauze that he'd need next.

I rolled my shoulders to ease the tension as Judy opened the
door. "Stop after this patient," she said. "Lunch is here."

When we finished the patient, I cleaned the instruments, the
dental chair, and the light. Disposing of my gown, goggles, and
gloves, I stepped outside the dental clinic and surveyed the scene
below me.

Crowds of people pressed like waves against the building,
trying to get relief from the unrelenting sun and their own

pressing needs. The construction crew strung tarps to offer partial shade.

The men in charge of traffic control radioed for help and struggled to make a path for us through the sea of people. After lunch, I took a few minutes to visit the eye clinic and check progress on the building the construction crew was raising. I peeped into the exam rooms and lab. I watched the pharmacy crew count out medication and fill prescriptions while Monty dressed a wound.

The transition from church to clinic never ceased to amaze me. Each trip, we arrived with a growing number of people. This year, there were volunteers from six churches in four states. We arrived, many of us having never met, with a mountain of boxes filled with medicine, equipment, and supplies.

One room became a storeroom for supplies. The choir loft was transformed into a pharmacy complete with shelves of medicine. Sunday school rooms became exam rooms. Classes were dismissed in the church's Christian school. Books and desks were stored. Those areas became the dental clinic and the eye clinic.

Even more amazing, within hours of the clinic opening, that diverse team of volunteers was functioning as a cohesive group. In the course of twenty-four hours, the church had been transformed into a clinic; strangers into a well-trained team.

I made my way to the sanctuary, where the patients who'd already seen a doctor and had their prescriptions filled met with members of the evangelism team. There, we birthed new souls into the kingdom of God, prayed for marriages to be restored, for demonic oppression to be removed, for fathers to return to their families, and for jobs and economic blessings.

That night, I dropped into bed and stared at the ceiling. I knew what we were doing was good. I also knew it wasn't God's best. I longed to see Jesus arise with healing in His wings—through the church. I ached for the day when, through prayer, teeth were filled, organs replaced, limbs made whole, and blind eyes received their sight.

I was hungry for God's glory to be manifest in our midst.

"Lord," I prayed, "why did You send us here as a medical mission?"

"You are a sign."

"A *sign*? I don't understand."

"This group is a sign I've given to the church. You are a physical manifestation of how the church is to be the church. It is a demonstration of unity that crosses denominational, doctrinal, and cultural boundaries. You are united to help not only the spiritual needs, but the physical needs as well. You are living stones. You are a sign."

Signs.

Those signs reminded me of a time when I was on voice rest. My doctor had given me strict orders not to speak. Just before Christmas, I still had shopping to do. My husband printed a notepad that introduced me and explained why I couldn't talk. There were lines for me to write out my request or question.

Notepad in hand, I arrived at a bicycle shop. I handed the salesman my pad on which I had written, *Hi, I'm on voice rest and can't speak. Could you please show me your bicycle helmets?*

The man read my note, looked up at me, and smiled. Then, turning, he shouted, "Hey, Joe! Got me a deaf-mute out here! I don't want to fool with it!" Then he turned back and smiled at me.

Sometimes I couldn't help but wonder if God might want to yell, "Hey, Jesus! Got me a bunch of deaf-mutes! I've tried talking to them, but they don't hear. I've written them letters, but they don't comprehend. Let's give them a sign!"

The Bible is full of recorded signs. Isaiah said, *"Here am I, and the children the LORD has given me. We are signs and symbols in Israel from the LORD Almighty"* (Isaiah 8:18).

I thought of Hosea. God told him to marry an adulterous wife so that he could be a sign and symbol to Israel that God would be faithful—even when they were not.

I wonder if Israel just thought Hosea was a bad judge of character?

Then there was Ezekiel. God told him to take tile and a metal pan to make a model of Jerusalem. Beside the model, he built a siege ramp. Then, tied in ropes, Ezekiel had to lie on his left side *in the road* for 390 days. Each day represented a year of Israel's iniquity. After 390 days in the road, God told him to turn on his right side for another 40 days representing the sins of Judah. (See Ezekiel 4:1–8.) Ezekiel spent a year and two months in the road as a sign to Israel!

Over the years, there have been many times when God asked me to do something I *really* didn't want to do. When I murmured, He said the one thing guaranteed to spur me toward obedience.

*"Have I asked **you** to lay in the road?"*

I know Him. That's not an idle threat. Besides, it puts the thing He asked me to do in the right perspective. It's usually not bad at all in comparison.

God is so faithful that He posts signs whether we read them or not. Here we were in Jamaica being a sign. I could only pray that somebody was watching.

We had a free day after we closed the clinic and before we flew home. I was shopping in a market in Montego Bay when I heard someone frantically calling my name.

"Melanie! Melanie!" Judy called. "You'll never guess who's here!"

"Who?" I asked, curious to see Judy wipe tears from her eyes.

"It's *him!* He's *here!*"

"*Who* is here?" I asked again, laughing.

"Winston!" she said, pointing.

Winston. None of us had seen him since our first trip to Jamaica, three years before. I turned and looked, first at his face. Then at his feet.

Winston still wore shoes.

Somehow, Judy found Don. Moments later, we celebrated a fond reunion. Winston's dreadlocks swung merrily under the stocking cap that he wore. We visited the shop where he sold the artwork he carved from wood. Don and I each found things that reminded us of something significant about Jamaica. I bought a wooden rooster that reminded me of the one that crowed outside the dental clinic at four each afternoon. Today, that rooster sits in a place of honor in my kitchen.

You might call it a sign—a reminder to pray for Jamaica.

Each time I look at it, I recall those last precious moments alone with Winston.

Introduce Me to him, Jesus whispered.

I did.

When the plane lifted off from the airport in Montego Bay, I leaned my head against the window to catch a last glimpse of Jamaica before we headed to open sea. I had a sad knowing that this trip marked the end of a season in my life. It seemed that my season had begun and ended with Winston.

Would God really send a group of people to be a physical sign of unity?

I thought of Isaiah, Ezekiel, and Hosea.

Yes, He would.

When the last visage of Jamaica disappeared from sight, I closed my eyes to rest.

I didn't think to ask the most obvious question.

Lord, what signs of our times have we failed to see?

With every deed you are sowing a seed, though the harvest you may not see.

—Ella Wheeler Wilcox

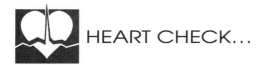 HEART CHECK...

It seems strange to think that God resorts to physical signs, but the Bible supports the fact that He does. While we shouldn't try to contrive them, neither should we ignore their existence. For me, the whole idea that God gives signs—like the stars that led wise men to Jesus—confirms how much we are loved and how desperately God is trying to communicate with us.

√ **Try doing a word search in the concordance to find the word** *sign* **in the Bible, and see what you learn.**

√ **What signs of the times has God shown to us? Might the following have been signs from God?**

- The fall of the Berlin Wall?
- The restoration of Israel as a nation?
- The discovery of the Dead Sea scrolls?

Father, I pray that You would open the eyes of my understanding and cause me to see the signs of the times. Give me wisdom and understanding to discern them correctly. I ask this in Jesus' name. Amen.

CHAPTER FIFTEEN

BLIND EYES

This is why I speak to them in parables: "Though seeing, they do not see; though hearing, they do not hear or understand."
—Matthew 13:13

There were signs. Everywhere. In retrospect, they were easy to read.

Except—we didn't.

Seeing, we did not see.

All you had to do was read a brief account of Oklahoma's history. Or take a scenic drive. The signs were there—some of them embossed on historical markers for the generations to read.

One site in the northeastern part of Oklahoma marked the final destination of the Cherokee Indians, whose homes in Georgia had been plundered and burned by local residents. Why? Because gold was discovered there.

The Supreme Court ruled that no one else had any claim to that land. Their ruling was ignored, and President Andrew Jackson refused to enforce it. Fifteen thousand Cherokees were evicted. During the fall and winter of 1838–39, with too little food and terrible suffering, they were driven, most of them on foot, to their new home in what is now Oklahoma.

Four thousand died along the Trail of Tears.

The history of Oklahoma had been a legacy of tears. The Cherokee joined Creek, Chickasaw, Choctaw, and Seminole tribes, who had all been forcibly removed from the southeastern United States by the government. They were herded to land that had been designated as a holding area for the Indian tribes. It began as a site for refugee camps, but they evolved into something closer to concentration camps.

Then, the land deeded to them was known as Indian Territory. After statehood, it was named Oklahoma. Two Choctaw words, *okla* meaning people, and *humma* meaning red, formed the name.

Oklahoma. Home of the red man.

No one gave a second thought to settling the Indians on this worthless land. After all, there was no gold in the plains. It took a while to discover there was another treasure.

Black gold.

Changing its mind again, the U.S. government took two million acres away from the tribes. It was up for grabs by white settlers and black freed men during the famous Land Run on April 22, 1889.[2] In a staggering number of strange coincidences, many of the families who claimed that land were stricken with infertility, insanity, and death.[3] It sounded like a curse. But curses were Old Testament stuff.

Weren't they?

Near the western border of Oklahoma, beside the Washita River, Black Kettle's band of peaceful Cheyenne camped where they'd been given permission by the U.S. government. They were the remnant who had survived the Sand Creek massacre in Colorado.

In November 1868, George Armstrong Custer and his regiment surprised the village. History books labeled that event "The Battle of the Washita."

Except it wasn't a battle.

It was a massacre.

Most of those who died were women and children.[4]

According to the Bible, Abel's blood cried to God from the ground. (See Genesis 4:10.) Many times the Bible warns that blood cries to God. The blood that soaked into Oklahoma soil in November of 1868 still cried. For years, parts of Oklahoma were so inhabited with outlaws the area was called "Badlands." Somehow, that name now seems prophetic.

In 1921 the worst race riot in the state's history occurred in Tulsa. Citizens burned out the black community, leaving three hundred known dead. Others ran for their lives, leaving the state never to return.

The next major sign occurred in 1930. It was called the Dust Bowl. The drought that hit lasted several years until the vegetation died. Spring winds literally blew the topsoil away, creating black blizzards that blocked the sun. In spite of the Great Depression and a scarcity of jobs nationwide, thousands of families were forced to abandon their homes—and the state—by the mid 1930s.

It was that dismal time in Oklahoma's history that sparked John Steinbeck's famous novel, *The Grapes of Wrath*. These days, I cannot think of that story without remembering that, according to Proverbs 26:2, *"the curse causeless shall not come"* (KJV).

What had caused this curse?

In Leviticus 26:40 God told Moses, *"But if they will confess their sins and the **sins of their fathers**..."* (emphasis added).

Could the drought that precipitated the Dust Bowl have been the result of unrepented sins, some of them committed by our ancestors?

Surely not, I reasoned. After all, God is just and merciful.

So just and merciful that He would withhold judgment for years? As members of the Oklahoma Concert of Prayer cried out to God for answers, He led us to the story of King David and the Gibeonites.

I flipped the pages of my Bible to read about the famine that struck Israel during King David's reign. The drought had been unrelenting for three years before David inquired of the Lord for the cause. *"The LORD said, 'It is on account of Saul and his blood-stained house; it is because he put the Gibeonites to death'"* (2 Samuel 21:1).

The Gibeonites lived in Israel's Promised Land. After the walls of Jericho had fallen, the Gibeonites realized they couldn't stand against the God of Israel. Their only hope was to trick the enemy into making a covenant with them.

So they lied.

They dressed in worn, ragged clothes. They poured wine into old wineskins. They carried molded bread. They convinced Joshua that they had traveled from a far country to be the Israelites' servants. According to the Bible,

> *The men of Israel sampled their provisions but did not inquire of the LORD. Then Joshua made a treaty of peace with them to let them live, and the leaders of the assembly ratified it by oath.* (Joshua 9:14–15)

Israel cut covenant, through a treaty, with their enemies—then they discovered the deceit.

But it was too late. Breaking a covenant *always* resulted in death.

Israel was stuck.

Years later, Saul *"in his zeal to the children of Israel and Judah"* (2 Samuel 21:2 KJV) slaughtered them.

More years passed as God's mercy waited for Israel to repent and restore. All the while, the blood of the Gibeonites cried to Him. When David realized the famine was due to a broken covenant, he knew that God would require both repentance and restoration to the descendants. He understood that atonement must be made and that Israel must have the blessings of the Gibeonite descendants to reverse the curse.

> *Wherefore David said unto the Gibeonites, What shall I do for you? and wherewith shall I make atonement that ye may bless the inheritance of the LORD?* (2 Samuel 21:3 KJV)

The Gibeonites required the blood of Saul's descendants. When the atonement had been made, they blessed Israel and the famine ended. Those Scriptures should have been a red flag signaling danger to this nation, and especially to Oklahoma. That famine was the result of one broken covenant. According to our government, treaties are the supreme law of the United States. Yet, that same federal government broke close to three hundred treaties with the American Indians. Hundreds more treaties were made with individual states and even Great Britain. None were fully kept. Many of those broken treaties involved land in Oklahoma.[5]

Like the Gibeonites, the United States had a covenant (treaty) with the Cheyenne who were massacred at the Washita. They had a covenant with the remnant of Cherokee who survived the Trail of Tears. They had covenants with the Choctaw and the Seminole. They had covenants with the Osage—whose deeded land in Oklahoma would prove to be one of the state's richest oil fields.

Those of us in the United States have an advantage over Saul's descendants. We already have an atonement sacrifice. Blood was spilled at the cross. But we failed to read the signs and repent. We failed to apply that precious blood. We failed to ask for a blessing.

Fifty years after the Dust Bowl, another devastation hit Oklahoma like an earthquake, with shock waves rippling throughout the nation. On July 2, 1982, a little bank located in the shadow of Penn Square Mall failed. I read of the event in the newspaper that day, and in the days to come. The bank's demise was of passing interest to most of us.

Seeing, we did not see.

Penn Square Bank had prospered during the oil and gas boom. It prospered so much that they had become a loan conduit to banks like Chase Manhattan, Continental Illinois, Seattle First, Northern Trust, and Michigan National.

The banking industry in Oklahoma collapsed like a house built out of cards. That financial failure was like a bomb-blast to the banking industry nationwide.

Was it another piece of bad luck in a long history of coincidences?

Or was it a rumbling of looming disaster following spilled blood and broken covenants?

We weren't asking questions like that back then. If we had, we would have realized that with broken covenants and bloodshed, the stronghold over this state wasn't a minor one.

It was death.

In August of 1986, Oklahoma made national news once again. Pat Sherrill, a disgruntled postal worker, walked into the Edmond Post Office with three pistols and one hundred rounds of ammunition hidden in a mailbag. At 7:02 that sultry morning, he began shooting, firing the last shot fifteen minutes later. Fourteen workers died and six were wounded before he shot himself, ending the third-largest mass murder in the nation's history up until that date.

Ken and I had moved to Edmond a mere five months before the shooting. Other tragedies were milestones along the path of destruction in the months leading up to the massacre. I remember well the continued shock as a series of murders plagued the town. That spring, a tornado wiped out one hundred Edmond homes.

Even then, I knew there was *something* we should be reading from these events. But we couldn't seem to put the pieces together to form a picture.

By 1994, there were definite signs of improvement. New construction had sprung up in a few select areas. While downtown Oklahoma City didn't bustle like it had during the oil boom, there were signs of life. Buildings that had sat vacant with "For Lease" signs in the windows long after Penn Square fell were now beginning to fill again.

One morning in June, I bolted upright in bed with a sheen of perspiration covering my face. I'd had a horrible dream. No, not a dream, it was a nightmare.

I dreamed that I was with a group in downtown Oklahoma City when a bomb exploded nearby...

The sound was deafening. Glass shards, pieces of brick, plaster, and metal shot through the air like shrapnel. We traveled north away from the bombsite, stepping carefully through the debris. The sidewalks were covered with blood. Blood splattered the streets.

There were three distinct bomb blasts, each closer than the last. Each blast left a huge crater. Afterward, there was an eerie silence. We stepped carefully through broken glass while dodging falling windows and walls...

My heart still hammered in my throat when I wrote the dream in my journal. Later, I typed it and asked other people to pray over it. The dream made no sense to me, but it left me feeling vulnerable.

Weeks and months passed while I struggled in prayer for the interpretation.

"Lord," I prayed, "I dreamed of a bomb in downtown Oklahoma City. What does the bomb symbolize?"

"A bomb."

"Lord, something is wrong," I said, chuckling. "I couldn't be hearing You right. I thought You said...*a bomb!*"

Dreams come true. Without that possibility, nature would not incite us to have them.
—*John Updike*

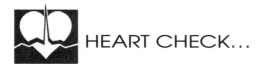 HEART CHECK…

The Father's heart is always turned toward His beloved children, and He speaks to us in many different ways. If only we could tune in to His frequency and understand God's language of love. The Bible says, *"Surely the Lord GOD will do nothing, but he revealeth his secret unto his servants the prophets"* (Amos 3:7 KJV).

In 1 Corinthians 4:1, Paul said, *"Let a man regard us in this manner, as servants of Christ, and stewards of the mysteries of God"* (NASB). In other words, God is determined to reveal mysteries and hidden things to His children.

One of the ways God communicates hidden things is through dreams. Does that mean every dream comes from God? No, it doesn't. Does it mean that we always understand God's messages and pray correctly? Assuredly not. But learning to communicate with God is undoubtedly our greatest purpose on earth. Communicating with God is like a slow dance. It's done heart to heart.

√ **In what ways do you know God has spoken to you?**
- Through the Bible
- Through spiritual leaders
- Through prophetic words
- Through dreams and visions
- Through a still, small voice
- Through signs

Father, please teach me the language of love. I want to know You. I ask this in Jesus' name. Amen

CHAPTER SIXTEEN

THE BOMB

Death has climbed in through our windows and
has entered our fortresses; it has cut off
the children from the streets and the
young men from the public squares.
—Jeremiah 9:21

I awoke early that morning, April 19, 1995. By five o'clock my husband, Ken, was awake too. All seemed well. Yet there was a strange tension in the air, the kind you feel just before an electrical storm here in Oklahoma. I slipped out of bed and pulled on my favorite blue robe. Outside my kitchen window, the morning sky was clear, cloudless.

There was a storm brewing.

But it wasn't the weather.

9:02 a.m. There was a deep rumble, like a beast arising from deep in the earth. *There's a natural gas explosion under my house!* I thought, too stunned to move. The house shook violently. The tall columns on my four poster bed waved in the air, lamps teetered precariously, and the chimes in our grandfather clock clanged against one another, sounding an eerie warning. Just when I thought the house would explode...it stopped.

Silence.

For the second time that morning, I looked outside for evidence of a tornado, a storm, *anything* that could explain what had just happened. Moments later, the silence was broken by the shrill ringing of the telephone.

"Melanie," my husband, Ken, said breathlessly, "we've been bombed."

Bombed.

I thought of my dream. The bomb wasn't spiritual symbolism. There was no symbolism to the blast that shook my house a full twelve miles away from downtown Oklahoma City. *A bomb in Oklahoma City?* I had thought, *How preposterous!*

That's probably the way a lot of people felt the day Noah closed the door to the ark and storm clouds gathered on the horizon. *Rain? Whoever heard of such a thing?*

Even though I hadn't grasped the dream's meaning, I was weak-kneed with gratitude that I had spent hours in prayer over the situation. Surely lives had been spared through my prayers and the prayers of others to whom God had shown the looming disaster. But it had not been averted. I swallowed hard, wondering how many lives had been lost.

"I'm all right," Ken assured me. "I can see it out my window—it looks like the Federal Building. Oh, Melanie...*Don!*"

One of our friends was a Secret Service agent in that building.

I shook my head as though to clear it. This wasn't a dream. We'd been bombed. And I *still* had trouble believing it.

"I don't know about the Kids," Ken continued.

The Kids! My heart froze. I knew Ken didn't mean our children, Heather and Lauren. They were safe at school here in Edmond. "The Kids" was his affectionate term for the *Russian*

Ballet on Ice troupe, a group of Russian figure skaters we'd recently come to know and love through a series of peculiarly divine connections. The skaters had been stranded in Oklahoma for seven months now and were living in the downtown YMCA.

Across the street from the Murrah Building!

"Ken, I've got to get down there," I gasped.

I thought about my young Russian friends. Strange, I'd never known them until recently. Yet the thought of one of them being hurt—or worse—sent numbing pain through my chest.

Each face flashed before me. I saw dark-haired Marina, the youngest at seventeen. I saw Inna's dancing eyes and expressive face. Gentle Alexi, so quiet, who always had a helping hand for others. I saw Anastasia at the amusement park the week before, pleading for "just one more" ride on the roller coaster. And Igor with his little Russian/English book. He'd been trying so hard to learn English. I saw Andrei, so serious. And Oksana's chiseled beauty.

One by one, I pictured each face and lifted their names to the Lord, until, finally, I saw Mikhail Belousov, the producer. His face, as always, weighted down by worry and responsibility.

I couldn't stand to lose one of them.

I saw flashing lights blocking the entrances to downtown. Because of my dream, I knew exactly how to get into the area. The bomb had been set off on Fifth Street. I entered at Tenth and pulled into the almost vacant parking lot of First Baptist Church.

Getting out of my car, I paused to look at the church where Ken and I had been married years before. So many of the old church's windows had been blown out by the blast that it looked like a snaggle-tooth caricature of its former stately self.

I started south on foot with the oddest sense of déjà vu. I felt like I'd stepped out of reality—and into my dream. Every last detail was exactly as I'd seen it.

The entire area looked like something out of a war movie. I paused to gape at the Journal Record Building located directly north of the Murrah Building. After years of housing their offices there, my husband's firm had moved a mere eight weeks earlier. An entire section of the roof was missing—and a gaping hole marked the spot where his law offices had been.

The remains of the Murrah Building and part of Fifth Street had been barricaded. Across the street from the YMCA, a temporary morgue had been set up. Around the corner, I found a crowd of people at the command center. There, looking bloody and beaten, stood Mikhail.

"Misha!" I shouted, calling his nickname. He was bleeding from lacerations all over his body, but the shocked look in his eyes concerned me most. Two of the skaters, Nikolai and Eteri, stood nearby wearing the same lost expression.

The troupe had been on the seventh floor of the YMCA when the bomb exploded. The large plate glass windows disintegrated into millions of missiles of flying glass. It sliced through them before they had time to move. The ceiling had collapsed on them. Water pipes burst, flooding the floors as they stumbled toward the stairway. They climbed down seven floors of debris to escape with what they were wearing.

Six of them had already been whisked away to hospitals.

"They've found a second device!" someone shouted.

The crowd exploded, running in every direction. In that split second I lost Nikolai and Eteri. I looked frantically for them, but they were invisible in the stampede. There was no way I could leave the area without them.

I didn't even know what direction to look. People were screaming, jostling, and running. Workers still fled the bombsite. I stood still in the midst of the panic and prayed.

After a few moments, and without conscious thought, I turned east and walked at a fast clip. I found myself a block away in an area that was almost deserted. God must have directed my steps, because there, huddled behind a building that appeared to be barely standing from the blast, knelt Nikolai and Eteri.

In the time it had taken me to find Nikolai and Eteri and wind our way back toward First Baptist Church, the Command Post had been moved and set up in the church parking lot. Fire trucks, police cars, other rescue vehicles surrounded my car.

I took one last look at the smoke that still rose from the ashes of downtown Oklahoma City. Traffic crawled as I drove out of the area and headed back to Edmond with my Russian friends. Finally, Nikolai spoke, struggling with the English words.

"Melanie, *why?*"

I shook my head. I didn't have words. Not in Russian. Not in English.

I delivered Nikolai and Eteri to the clubhouse that an apartment complex had opened to the troupe. Twenty skaters were gathered around the television, watching in horror the replays of what they'd just escaped.

I drove back downtown to check on the skaters still in hospitals.

By five o'clock that afternoon, the last skater was released from the hospital. The other five had already been released and were in Edmond with the rest of the group.

They were all wounded. They had only the bloody clothes they wore. They didn't have combs, toothbrushes, or bottles of shampoo. They were crowded into one room with a sofa, a small table, and four kitchen chairs.

They needed a home.

They needed a healing touch.

They needed intensive caring.

Ken and I invited them to stay with us.

By evening there was a steady stream of people bringing food, pillows, blankets, and air mattresses into our house. The skaters gathered in the family room in front of the television. Instead of watching the news, my children turned on video games. *Good,* I thought, *they don't need to see the bomb scene over and over. And neither do my children.*

Ken and I stole a few minutes to talk privately. "Don's alive," he said.

"Thank God!"

"I missed it by six minutes," Ken said.

"You *what?*"

"I was in front of the Murrah Building six minutes before it exploded."

Our eyes met. We looked at one another in the longest, most profound silence of our marriage. Then we fell into one another's arms.

Heather, Lauren, and the dog slept in our room, because their rooms were filled with people. When the house finally settled down, it felt cozy, warm...and safe.

Everyone in Oklahoma City felt safe last night.

I lay in bed and thought about the three blasts in my dream. Had Satan planned three different bombs? I couldn't know for sure. But already the reports were streaming in from all over town and beyond. God had warned many people. Most, like me, had trouble taking the bomb warnings as literal.

It was difficult for an infinite God to intercede through finite minds.

The worst terrorist act ever committed on U.S. soil to that date had happened here. *Why?* I wondered, falling into a dreamless sleep.

Late evening became my favorite time of day. The phone stopped ringing, reporters and cameramen went to their hotels, and my Russian guests assembled in the family room to watch movies. Their favorites were not the real-life dramas, but the animated films I had bought for my children. I loved to stand in the doorway—not to watch the movies—just to hear their laughter. Although they couldn't understand the words, they thrilled at the antics of cartoon kings and princes whose adventures always ended in triumph, and whose dreams always came true.

But when their laughter stopped, many times they gathered in the kitchen to talk. What was going to happen to them? Would they ever get their skates from the YMCA? Without skates, they had no future. No hope at all.

A visiting Russian pastor from St. Petersburg, Nikki Nikkitin, arrived at my house like a breath of fresh air. The skaters flocked to him, chattering in their own language. Pastor Nikki sat on the hearth and opened a Russian Bible. He spent hours teaching them about God and reading them Scripture. He explained God's plan to redeem mankind through the cross. Fifteen heads bowed in prayer. Fifteen hearts believed.

Two days later, the Labor Department sent a special team of workers dressed in protective gear into the asbestos-strewn ruins of the YMCA to retrieve what had not been destroyed. Twenty Russians cheered when they saw boxes of their belongings. But the cheering stopped suddenly when the first pair of skates was lifted from the box.

The blades were pitted with rust, the boots soggy and soft from standing water. Mentally, I calculated the cost of professional skates. How could they ever replace all twenty pair? The future of *Russian Ballet on Ice* had gone up in smoke with a bomb blast.

I remembered the five performances I'd seen in Oklahoma City. The beauty had tugged my heart. How could there *not* be other performances, other tours?

The next day, someone donated seven apartments rent-free for two months. We drove Misha to look at the apartments.

"You think," he said quietly, pointing toward heaven, "God?"

"Yes," I said, grinning. "I think God did this."

The next week we learned that Reidell, one of the leading manufacturers of skates, offered to sell twenty pairs of skates at cost. Kenneth Copeland Ministries purchased them.

When a translator announced the news to the troupe, they blinked in stunned silence. Then, Marina slipped to the kitchen. Eyes flashing, she jumped for joy. Midair, she whispered one word. *"Skates!"*

Only God could bring beauty from the ashes of this tragedy.

With generous help from Southern Nazarene University, some of the skaters flew home to Russia. Others joined traveling ice shows. These days, I get occasional cards from Japan, the Philippines, Egypt, Europe—wherever they may be performing pirouettes on ice.

I wished that God could heal this city and state as quickly. But the parts had been broken in too many pieces for a quick fix. Still, every day Clark Kent-type men became heroes. People crawled into the shifting crater to dig for bodies. People nursed the wounded and cradled the dying. Some identified bodies and manned morgues. Others, in the hospital waiting rooms, handed out quarters for phone calls, offered coffee, juice, and food. Restaurants fed rescue workers free day after day. Volunteers washed their clothes, made their cots, and left them notes and treats.

Perhaps the most profound change occurred when churches from every denomination drew together to pray for this state and nation. Through the Oklahoma Concert of Prayer, they set up watchmen on the walls to pray, as well as a system to quickly distribute prayer concerns to church leaders in the city and across the state. Now warning dreams like the one I had could be immediately distributed to key spiritual leaders.

April 19, 1995 was the darkest day in Oklahoma's history.

It was also her finest hour.

It proved one thing beyond a shadow of a doubt.

The church survived the blast.

> *A* man should not leave this earth with unfinished business. He should live each day as if it was a pre-flight check. He should ask each morning, am I prepared to lift-off?
> —*Diane Frolov &*
> *Andrew Schneider*

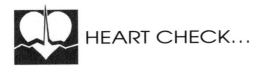 HEART CHECK...

We've all been blindsided by the enemy at different times in our lives. Your marriage my have suffered a fatal blow. You may have encountered enemy fire on the ladder to career success. Like the Russian skaters, you might have just been in the wrong place at the wrong time. If we got to choose all the days of our lives, we would never choose to be in harm's way. But when our plans get bombed, we do have a choice in our response.

We can get bitter.

Or we can get better.

Which option you take may well depend on how deeply you believe one crucial revelation: *God cares intensely for you.*

√ **Look back over the situations where you've been blindsided by the enemy.**

- List all the ways that God cared intensively for you before, during, and after that crisis in your life.
- What do you trust Him to resurrect in your life?

√ **If you choose to get better instead of bitter, God can use you to provide intensive caring to a hurting world. Isaiah listed the requirements for this elite group:**

- Loose the bonds of wickedness.
- Undo the heavy burdens.
- Let the oppressed go free.
- Break every yoke.
- Share your bread with the hungry.
- Bring to your house the poor who are cast out.
- Cover the naked when you see him.

- Take away the pointing of the finger, and speaking wickedness.
- Extend your soul to the hungry.
- Satisfy the afflicted soul (Isaiah 58:6–10 NKJV).

Father, teach me to live the fast that Isaiah taught.
Cause me to be qualified to care for a hurting world,
and give me Your heart of compassion. I ask this in
Jesus' name. Amen.

Then your light shall dawn in the darkness, and your dark-
ness shall be as the noonday. The Lord will guide you continu-
ally, and satisfy your soul in drought, and strengthen your
bones; you shall be like a watered garden, and like a spring of
water, whose waters do not fail. Those from among you shall
build the old waste places; you shall raise up the foundations
of many generations; and you shall be called the Repairer of
the Breach, the Restorer of Streets to Dwell In.

(Isaiah 58:10–12 NKJV)

CHAPTER SEVENTEEN

INTENSIVE CARING FOR A HURTING WORLD

Nations are in an uproar, kingdoms fall;
he lifts his voice, the earth melts.
—Psalm 46:6

*T*he air carried a hint of fall on September 11, 2001, and New York City woke to the promise of a beautiful day. Radios played familiar strains as families offered hurried good-byes that no one suspected would be forever. Children shrugged on backpacks and stuffed sandwiches into their lunch boxes. Mothers ran back to plug in the slow cooker for dinner before racing to the power meeting ahead. Men hustled down the subway entrance with steaming cups of coffee in one hand and newspapers in the other. Taxicabs honked at other drivers, train whistles sounded an alarm, and phones rang while delis did a brisk business.

It was just another day in New York City.

Or so it seemed.

The whole world paused to watch airliners fly into the twin towers of the World Trade Center. America lost her innocence when the massive steel structures imploded upon themselves.

Who could have imagined a hijacked airliner filled with innocent people flying into the Pentagon, the symbol of our military strength?

I clicked off the nightly news, but I couldn't click off the images that replayed on the screen of my mind. The home of the brave was under siege. Biological weapons invaded media offices, corporate headquarters, and even the inner chambers of our government. Most thinking people knew that what happened in America on 9/11 stemmed from a world in crisis. There was no doubt about it in my mind—the nations of the world were being shaken through war and terrorism.

There may have never been a time in history when national boundaries changed so rapidly that mapmakers couldn't keep abreast of the revisions. Nor when kingdoms fell as quickly as the Berlin Wall had crumbled. Now, the Japanese economy, an anchor in the world's banking system, teetered precariously as the Yen dropped in value. Unlike Penn Square Bank, whose fall toppled banks throughout the United States, a sudden demise in the Japanese Yen threatened the economic future of nations.

Everything that isn't grounded firmly in God and His Word is sinkable, I thought, kneeling to pray.

I knew there had been doomsayers predicting these events, and worse, for years. Some, even Christians, had stockpiled food and money. Others had built fortresses in the mountains. Few people, Christian or atheist, doubted that there was a shaking ahead.

To me, the thought of hiding from looming disaster seemed laughable. Recently, I'd read about the number of nuclear missiles that disappeared from the Soviet Union's arsenal when that nation splintered like shattered glass.

As far as I could tell, there was no place to run. No place to hide.

Except one—in Him. The psalmist calls it the *"secret place of the Most High"* (Psalm 91:1 NKJV).

Besides, many of the ills that plagued our world were the direct result of Christians hiding their heads in the sand. It was time to stand up and be counted. More to the point, it was time to kneel down, repent, and wield the sword of the Spirit over the nations.

There are judgments coming to the nations of the world that we cannot stop. The Bible describes a judgment where each nation will be ruled as sheep or goats. We can't stop that judgment from coming, but we can—and must—use the authority of our prayers to affect the outcome.

I recall reading about a Christian woman, who at God's direction, moved into a house directly over a fault line in California. For years she knelt over that fault and prayed for peace and quiet.

That, I believe, is the spiritual picture of how we, as Christians, must nurse this dying world. To understand our responsibility, it's important to look to Scripture. In Genesis, God created the earth and all its fullness and gave dominion over it to man.

We find this authority granted in the Garden of Eden:

Then God blessed them, and God said to them, "Be fruitful and multiply; fill the earth and subdue it; have dominion over the fish of the sea, over the birds of the air, and over every living thing that moves on the earth." (Genesis 1:28 NKJV)

But Adam committed high treason and sinned against God by eating of the forbidden tree. At that time, a change occurred in authority. According to 2 Corinthians 4:4 KJV, Satan became the *"god of this world."* Because of Adam's sin, Satan gained dominion.

It wasn't until the sinless Son of God came to earth that He gained authority. We see this in the following Scriptures:

My Father has given me authority over everything.
(Matthew 11:27 NLT)

Jesus came and told His disciples, "I have been given complete authority in heaven and on earth." (Matthew 28:18 NLT)

The Father loves his Son, and he has given him authority over everything. (John 3:35 NLT)

Then Jesus came and spoke to them, saying, "All authority has been given to Me in heaven and on earth."
(Matthew 28:18 NKJV)

Jesus passed His authority on to His disciples:

Then He called His twelve disciples together and gave them power and authority over all demons, and to cure diseases.
(Luke 9:1 NKJV)

With my authority, take this message of repentance to all the nations, beginning in Jerusalem: "There is forgiveness of sins for all who turn to me." (Luke 24:47 NLT)

Behold, I give you the authority to trample on serpents and scorpions, and over all the power of the enemy, and nothing shall by any means hurt you. (Luke 10:19 NKJV)

Jesus is the head of the church; we are His body.

There is a war in the heavenlies, and the outcome is up to us. Satan is doing everything in his limited power to keep control of the earth. Jesus bought back the world through His death on the cross. You and I are called to enforce that victory.

Today, a limitless God is limited only by the prayers we pray—or fail to pray.

The fall of the Berlin Wall was a sign and a wonder to the world. Yet that wall did not fall except through prayer. There is no way of knowing, this side of heaven, how many people made pilgrimages there to pray. There were doubtless hundreds if not thousands. Countless others around the world knelt before the throne of God to pray it down. When the Lord's cup was full of those prayers, nothing on earth could have kept it standing.

I heard recently of an awakening that broke out affecting a whole country. Many people believe it was the direct result of one American child who set herself to pray for that nation daily for two years. Perhaps that is why Jesus said we should become like little children. Childlike faith in prayer can change the course of nations.

I'm convinced that at the end of this age God's heroes will be men, women, boys, and girls who no one on earth remembers. Most will be anonymous people who did nothing outstanding in their lives.

Except pray.

Alone in their prayer closets, they prayed over the nations of the world. Nations rose and fell in response to their prayers.

Because I understand the importance of winning nations to the Lord, I was somewhat surprised when He instructed Ken and me to join a church whose vision was to win our city.

"Why pray for cities when nations are at stake?" I asked the Lord.

In answer, He took me in the Bible to the scriptural picture of *His* order in evangelism. It was the last thing He spoke to His disciples before He ascended into heaven.

But ye shall receive power, after that the Holy Ghost is come upon you: and ye shall be witnesses unto me both in Jerusalem, and in all Judaea, and in Samaria, and unto the uttermost part of the earth. (Acts 1:8 KJV)

Notice the order. Jesus directed them to go first to Jerusalem, then to Judaea, then Samaria, and finally to the world.

"*No church will fulfill her call to the nations if she refuses to fulfill the call to her city,*" the Lord said.

The Lord directed me to Acts 1:4:

On one occasion, while he was eating with them, he gave them this command: "Do not leave Jerusalem, but wait for the gift my Father promised, which you have heard me speak about."

As I meditated on this passage, I realized that although Jesus was speaking directly to the church of that day, He was also speaking to us today. When those who obeyed His instruction to wait in Jerusalem received what the Father had promised, three thousand were added to their number in one day!

Waiting in unity on the Lord in Jerusalem brought great multiplication to the church. Those greater numbers went to Judaea and multiplied again. Even greater numbers went to Samaria and then to the world.

I am convinced that each of us is responsible to pray over the nations of the world—and that we will be held accountable for those prayers before God. But to win the world, we must wait on God in unity in our own Jerusalem—or Oklahoma City, Fort Worth, New York City, Los Angeles, Chicago, Detroit, Hong

Kong, Beijing, Honolulu, Singapore, St. Petersburg, and cities around the world.

I have put my finger on the pulse of the nations through prayer, and I can tell you that this world is in critical condition. It is critical that we care enough—to pray.

> *War* is much too serious a matter to be entrusted to the military.
>
> —*Georges Clemenceau*

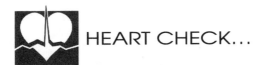 HEART CHECK...

I believe that you and I are blessed to live in this hour of history. We are living in the last days when God's clock is ticking as we spin toward eternity. A great crowd of heavenly witnesses have gathered around to watch the outcome of the war over the precious harvest of the world. It is possible for you to live in an uncertain world with the certainty that your life on earth makes an eternal difference.

All of heaven is poised to hear your voice.

√ **What nation of the world has God placed on your heart?**
√ **Are you willing to watch over that nation in prayer?**
√ **God will assuredly do His part. Are you willing to do yours?**

Father, thank You for choosing me to live in these historic times. Give me grace to watch and pray effectively over a wounded and dying world. Give me the nations for my inheritance. Thank You. I pray this in Jesus' name. Amen.

CHAPTER EIGHTEEN

INCOMING!

You have not strengthened the weak or healed the sick or bound up the injured. You have not brought back the strays or searched for the lost.
—Ezekiel 34:4

I sank onto the sofa next to Ken late one evening and observed the ritual he called watching television. I watched with fascination as a rhythmic spasm of Ken's thumb clicked through channels as program after program flashed across the screen only to disappear moments later.

Granted, there wasn't much worth watching, but what was it about some men and their remote control?

On the rare evenings that Ken did watch a program from beginning to end, he preferred real-life dramas: cops and robbers or serious medical shows.

Not me.

Nursing, both physical and spiritual, left me intense and serious about life. If I wanted entertainment, I preferred comic relief. Ken paused to watch a few minutes of a show portraying an emergency room scene. I looked away. I did not enjoy those programs.

First, most of them were medically inane. I remembered one of the last serious medical shows I'd watched years before. A man with an apparent heart attack arrived in the emergency room. He was transferred to a gurney and two orderlies raced down a hospital corridor with him. A doctor ran alongside listening to the man's heart sounds.

Really. As though he could hear those quiet sounds through all that clatter! Well, okay, maybe that one *was* comic relief, but that hadn't been the producer's plan. When scenes were done realistically, I walked away feeling like I'd been at work for an hour.

Stressful work.

Ken clicked to a new channel, and I heard the familiar strains from the theme song of *M*A*S*H.* Even before I glanced at the screen, I heard the drone of a helicopter bringing more wounded to the 4077.

I knew that if I let myself watch it for even a few minutes, I'd be hooked. *M*A*S*H* was one of the few shows on television that I had always enjoyed. Although I never thought to turn it on and purposely watch it, when the reruns came on late at night during Ken's ritual, I could rarely resist it.

In deference to me, Ken somehow managed to control his remote control hand until commercials, when he frantically clicked through every channel. I never fully understood what it was about *M*A*S*H* that appealed to me. Perhaps it was the wacky humor the characters used to handle their stress. Perhaps it was how very *human* they were in the midst of their heroics.

One show in particular haunts me to this day. The primary character was Major Margaret "Hot Lips" Hoolihan—a woman who gave nurses everywhere a bad name. Margaret was so war-hardened that she witnessed the atrocities with hardly a second glance. She certainly had no patience with nurses who wept, shook, or showed signs of strain.

That is, until the day the stray dog she'd been feeding was hit by a jeep. Major Hoolihan unwound like a broken clock. The strange thing was that the moment the jeep hit the dog, *my* emotions unwound as well. I knew it was fiction, but my reaction was not. I doubled over holding myself like I was falling apart and wept in agony.

During all those years I'd worked in intensive care, like Major Hoolihan's character, I'd learned to dismiss the atrocities I saw: the five-year-old boy, brain dead with purple bruises around his neck where his father strangled him with a pair of nylons.

Or the time I took care of a twenty-eight-year-old man who'd carried a lantern into his storm cellar during a tornado warning. He didn't know there was a gas leak until the explosion burned him past recognition.

Dressed in gown, mask, and gloves, I gently lifted his left hand to check the dressings over his IV. One moment his hand was in mine; the next it slipped to the bed. That is, the bones, ligaments, and muscles slipped to the bed. His skin and fingernails lay in my hand like a glove someone had discarded.

Dear God!

I stared at it in horror, then saw the achingly blue eyes that looked up at me from a face that no longer appeared human. Gasping for air, I glanced up at the lone window in the isolation room. There, staring back at me were a pair of deep blue eyes.

My patient's identical twin brother.

Our eyes locked in agony.

I wanted to tear the gown and mask off and run, sobbing, from that hospital never to return. I wanted my own innocence back. I wanted never to have seen or felt what I'd just experienced. I didn't want to know about those kinds of tragedies.

But I did know.

I had experienced it.

I couldn't run.

The man needed someone to tend him gently until he drew his last ragged breath. That's all I could give him. It was one of the hardest things I ever did, giving myself that way. I choked back my feelings. Swallowed them hard. Dismissed them. And did what had to be done.

But many times driving home from work, I'd see a dog lying broken beside the road. Immediately, sorrow would well up in me so deep that I'd want to scream in agony, too blinded by tears to see the road ahead.

I didn't tell people of my strange malady. Psychiatrists would probably have labeled it some kind of posttraumatic stress syndrome. At the very least, they would tell me I projected all the grief I couldn't express at work onto dead animals. Intellectually, I knew that was true. Emotionally, it seemed too simple.

Even now, years later, I can't look at an animal beside the road. It costs me too dearly. Deer heads mounted on walls make me nauseous. I shake at the site of a bearskin rug.

God, how I hate death.

When will it be finished?

Will death's hunger ever be satisfied?

The first time I came emotionally unwound watching a jeep hit Major Hoolihan's dog, I felt strangely comforted when I stopped crying. Someone who wrote that script *knew*. They understood. Someone out there had lived where I was living.

I was not alone.

There were many things about *M*A*S*H* that I identified with. One of the most important was what happened when the hum of helicopters sounded on the horizon and loud speakers warned the unit, "Incoming!"

Until that moment, it was life as usual: bickering, petty jealousy, and practical jokes. But the moment the alarm was sounded for incoming wounded, everything else in the camp stopped. To a person, they rallied under the hardest of circumstances to save lives. For most of them, it didn't matter if the victim was friend or enemy—they worked to save him.

And fought the *real* enemy—death.

Over the years, I've noticed many similarities between that piece of fiction and real-life intensive care, even in the church. In a magazine interview, Steve Hill, an evangelist in the Brownsville Assembly of God revival that occurred in Pensacola, Florida, said:

> The church in the United States and other parts of the world has been in an intensive care unit. It's lost its life; you can barely hear a pulse. But through the renewal, the Lord is reviving the church—the whole body of Christ, not just individuals here and there.
>
> On the heels of revival, then, comes spiritual awakening. An awakening moves past the local body of believers and goes into the community. Drug addicts, alcoholics, prostitutes, businessmen, and others who have never known the Lord start getting saved. The church goes into the highways and byways and compels people to come in.[6]

If the church has been in intensive care—and we have—it is time for us to crawl up on the surgical table and allow our hearts to be newly circumcised. It is time for the church to turn to the

Great Physician and cry out for healing. Because now it's time for the church to *become* an intensive care unit for a sick and dying world.

These days, I let my hatred of death drive me to prayer. Romans 8:22–23 says,

We know that the whole creation has been groaning as in the pains of childbirth right up to the present time. Not only so, but we ourselves, who have the firstfruits of the Spirit, groan inwardly as we wait eagerly for our adoption as sons, the redemption of our bodies.

Through prayer, I join the groaning of *all creation* awaiting full redemption.

There is a glorious day coming when we will fully put off the old man and put on the new man. We will do it as easily as my patient slipped out of his earthbound hand. Then, death, where will be your sting? Grave, where will be your victory?

Until then, there is work to be done. Those of us who are fortunate enough to be alive in this hour of history were brought to earth for such a time as this.

You see, the church is coming of age.

Listen carefully, and you'll hear the hum of helicopters on the horizon.

You'll hear the Holy Spirit sounding an alarm to the church.

"INCOMING!"

ENDNOTES

1   Norman Grubb, *Rees Howells: Intercessor* (Fort Washington, Penn.: CLC Publications, 1952), 30.

2   Encyclopedia Britannica, 15th ed., sv "Oklahoma."

3   Cindy Jacobs, message to Oklahoma Concert of Prayer, Church on the Rock, OK, April 1996.

4   U.S. Department of the Interior, Battle of the Washita Historical Site Brochure, Cheyenne, OK.

5   International Reconciliation Coalition/Indigenous People, Jean Steffenson, President, Castle Rock, CO.

6   Steve Hill, "A Burden for the Lost," *Charisma,* (July 1997): 52.

ABOUT THE AUTHOR

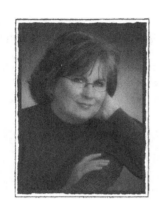

A former intensive care nurse, Melanie Hemry traded in her stethoscope for a computer and now writes poignant true-life stories, many of which are set in intensive care. A winner of the coveted *Guideposts* Writing Contest, Melanie's stories have warmed the hearts of readers around the world. She holds a bachelor of science in nursing from the University of Central Oklahoma and a master's degree in practical ministry from Wagner Leadership Institute in Colorado Springs.

In addition to having written *A Healing Touch* and dozens of stories for *Guideposts*, Melanie is a regular feature-article contributor to the *Believer's Voice of Victory* magazine with nearly 500,000 readers. She and co-author Gina Lynnes have collaborated on a series of inspirational gift books about the miraculous power of God's anointing: *Anointing for Healing, Anointing for Children, Anointing for Loved Ones' Salvation,* and *Anointing for Protection.*

Melanie is also a popular speaker for church groups and women's retreats. She can be reached at www.melaniehemry.com.

Anointing for Healing
Melanie Hemry & Gina Lynnes

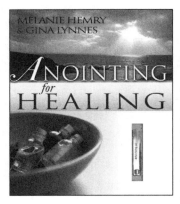

Melanie Hemry and Gina Lynnes share personal experiences and researched testimonies of people miraculously healed by a powerful God who still works in our lives today. Even when the situation was seemingly hopeless, God intervened to heal. This combination of amazing stories and powerful Scripture will have you in awe and wonder over the greatness and love of God. You will learn the significance of anointing oil when praying for healing, discover how to pray effectively, and find inspiration for your Christian walk. This book is what you need to break through to your healing experience.

ISBN: 978-0-88368-687-4 • Gift • 176 pages

Anointing for Children
Melanie Hemry & Gina Lynnes

The devil is out to get our children. Most of us have already figured that out. What we need to know is how to keep them out of his hands. Find out how other determined parents have done it. Discover the scriptural truths that inspired them and witness the miracles that happened in their children's lives as they stepped out in faith on God's Word. Whether you're hoping to have a baby, needing healing for your child, or praying for a prodigal to come home, *Anointing for Children* has a message of hope and faith for you.

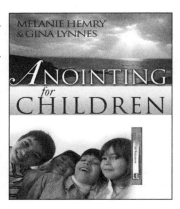

ISBN: 978-0-88368-686-7 • Gift • 192 pages

www.whitakerhouse.com

Anointing for Protection
Melanie Hemry & Gina Lynnes

God has the power to protect His people from danger. Eloise Wright proved it in a Dallas parking lot when a kidnapper locked her at gunpoint in the trunk of her car. Eloise's astounding story, along with the testimonies of other believers who faced hair-raising disasters in faith and miraculously survived them unharmed, are a thrilling reminder that the God of the Bible is still guarding His people today. Find out how you can build your life on God's promises of protection so that you too can live in supernatural security even in the most dangerous of times.

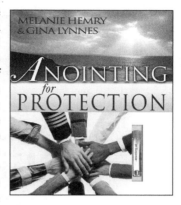

ISBN: 978-0-88368-689-8 • Gift • 208 pages

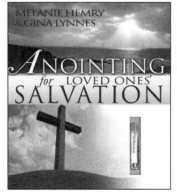

Anointing for Loved Ones' Salvation
Melanie Hemry & Gina Lynnes

Some people need a Damascus road experience—a supernatural manifestation of the Holy Spirit, a sign or a wonder like those in the book of Acts—to bring them out of darkness and into the light. But do such things still happen today? Absolutely. These thrilling stories prove it. Full of real-life testimonies told by those who have been dramatically saved, this book abounds with clear, scriptural promises that will inspire you to pray for lost loved ones with fresh fervor and faith. It will help keep you on your knees until the victory is won.

ISBN: 978-0-88368-688-1 • Gift • 192 pages

WHITAKER HOUSE

www.whitakerhouse.com

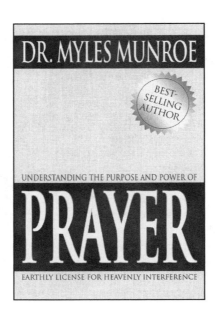

Understanding the Purpose and Power of Prayer
Dr. Myles Munroe

All that God is—and all that God has—may be received through prayer. Everything you need to fulfill your purpose on earth is available to you through prayer. The biblically based, time-tested principles presented here by Dr. Myles Munroe will ignite and transform the way you pray. Be prepared to enter into a new dimension of faith, a deeper revelation of God's love, and a renewed understanding that you can pray—and receive results.

ISBN: 978-0-88368-442-9 • Trade • 240 pages

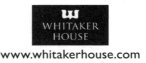

WHITAKER
HOUSE

www.whitakerhouse.com